Y0-EDX-029
COLL
LIBRARY
JAN 1 6 1985
DALLAS, PENNSYLVANIA

HOSPITAL ORIENTATION HANDBOOK

for Nurses and Allied Health Professionals

Ann Haggard, R.N., M.S., Ph.D.
Huntington Memorial Hospital
Pasadena, California

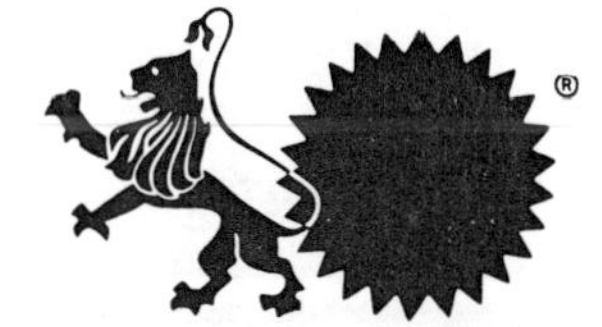

AN ASPEN PUBLICATION®
Aspen Systems Corporation
Rockville, Maryland
Royal Tunbridge Wells
1984

Library of Congress Cataloging in Publication Data

Haggard, Ann.
Hospital orientation handbook for nurses and allied health professionals.

Bibliography: p. 273
Includes index.
1. Hospitals—Staff—In-service training. 2. Nurses—In-service training. 3. Allied health personnel—In-service training. I. Title
[DNLM: 1. Personnel Administration, Hospital. 2. Personnel, Hospital—education. WX 159 H145h]
RA972.5.H28 1984 610′.715 84-6514
ISBN: 0-89443-589-2

Publisher: John R. Marozsan
Associate Publisher: Jack W. Knowles, Jr.
Editorial Director: N. Darlene Como
Executive Managing Editor: Margot G. Raphael
Managing Editor: M. Eileen Higgins
Editorial Services: Ruth M. McKendry
Printing and Manufacturing: Debbie Collins

Library of Congress Catalog Card Number: 84-6514
ISBN: 0-89443-589-2

Printed in the United States of America

1 2 3 4 5

To my parents . . .
with gratitude

Table of Contents

Preface

When I went into hospital education, one of my first duties was to conduct orientation classes. Since I had never done it before, I headed to the literature for help. What I found were a few journal articles, but what I wanted was a comprehensive reference that would explain the entire process in detail and offer some new ideas on how to do it.

Without such help, I learned by trial and error. Eventually, I was made orientation coordinator of a 565-bed hospital with over 2,500 employees, conducting large orientation classes of many different types. But I never stopped looking for that comprehensive reference.

This book is the one I was trying to find. In it I have taken the research, wisdom, and advice of as many professional educators as I could find and combined it with my own experience to put together a complete handbook on orienting hospital employees. The purpose of this book is to help instructors to

- Systematically identify and analyze learning needs
- Compose pertinent, clearly stated objectives
- Apply the principles of adult education to the orientation process
- Organize and schedule instruction so that effective and efficient learning occurs
- Use a variety of instructional methods, techniques, and strategies
- Use a range of resources and media during orientation presentations
- Provide effective follow-up and reinforcement to orientees in the clinical areas
- Employ evaluation techniques to assess orientees' achievement and to judge the effectiveness of the orientation process

Do you hate the very sound of the word ''orientation''? For a hospital instructor orientation can come to be dreaded—almost as much as it's dreaded by the orientees. Why? Why is orientation perceived by both teachers and audience as a boring ordeal to be lived through?

Let's glance over some typical evaluations of an orientation program: ''Lectures are boring'' . . . "Redundant information" . . . "Dull speaker" . . . "Too long to sit" . . . etc., etc. The instructor struggles with the impulse to shout ''*You* try to make it interesting!''

Sitting in class listening to lectures about required information such as charting and infection control seems expressly designed to put people to sleep. Don't despair. There are a number of tested strategies you can use to make orientation not only interesting but absorbing. The more you can involve participants in the content, the more of the information they will remember and be able to apply to patient care. And that's really what it's all about, isn't it?

This book is designed to cover the subject of orientation comprehensively, to offer specific techniques that any instructor can adapt for use in whatever hospital environment is available. Whether your institution is a multiservice facility with hundreds of beds and a large education budget or a small rural hospital with no budget at all, you can take the ideas and make them work for you.

Chapter 1 offers a brief overview of the orientation process, including how orientation got started and why it became so important to hospitals and employees alike. It also supplies some cost analysis data that you (as well as your administrators) may find surprising and goes through some recent research on the stages of orientation and what should be expected from them.

Chapter 2 explores what subjects should be covered in orientation and how this decision can be made in your institution. It's not something that should be left to chance or tradition. Setting priorities for selection and order of content is the vital first step in making your orientation an important part of a new employee's experience.

Chapter 3 covers orientation objectives, a subject that everyone gives lip service to but few actually spend much time on. Carefully designed objectives, stated in behavioral terms, will help you decide what should be included and how it should be presented, so don't skip this part.

Chapter 4 explores different methods of actually presenting the content. Will participants incorporate vital information if it's presented in a series of lectures? We all know the answer to that: no way. No matter how interesting a speaker the instructor may be, the more teaching strategies that are used, the more attention the information will get. Beginning with a brief discussion of the principles of adult education, this section goes through many different ways of presenting content. Sample class outlines and different examples of how these varied methods are actually used in orientation follow.

Chapters 5 through 7 present the specifics of orienting allied personnel (employees who do not work in nursing areas). Only recently have they received much attention from hospital education, but the orientation of these employees is just as vital as the orientation of the nursing staff.

Chapters 8 and 9 detail classroom and clinical components of nursing orientation, the area where most instructors become "burned out." These chapters will present some new ideas and techniques to revitalize the exhausted imagination.

Chapter 10 goes into the relatively new but fast-growing area of new graduate orientation. Since Marlene Kramer's findings about Reality Shock, most hospitals try to prepare new graduate nurses for the role of staff nurse, with varying degrees of success. This section will review the types of programs and give some specific strategies that can ease this difficult transition.

Chapter 11 covers orientation in the various specialty areas. Whether critical care, maternal-child health, or a fairly new specialty such as neonatal intensive care, each area has esoteric knowledge and skills that must be mastered by nurses who wish to work there. How this information is covered can have vital importance for both patients and practitioners.

Chapter 12 delves into the orientation of nurse attendants, orderlies, and unit secretaries. Should the hospital train its own or should it hire only experienced people and offer an orientation program similar to that for nurses? Both alternatives are explored—you make the final decision.

Chapter 13 presents methods of evaluating orientees. Important clues about future performance can be picked up during orientation. Do you have a system for identifying crucial incidents and communicating them to the orientee's manager? Such a system could mean the difference between a safe practitioner and a threat to patients.

Chapter 14 considers the evaluation of the orientation program itself. Can you prove that your program made a difference? This is probably the most difficult part of any educational endeavor.

Chapter 15 addresses the problem of proving the cost effectiveness of orientation, a task some say is impossible. It also goes in for a spot of crystal-ball gazing into the future of orientation and where we go from here. The final direction that the program takes will ultimately depend on you.

Throughout this book I will try to give you information that is usable—techniques that have proven themselves under actual classroom conditions. The aim is to give you a reference that you can return to for tips to help revise your programs and lessen the stress associated with teaching this most important aspect of staff development.

And now, on to ORIENTATION!

Ann Haggard

Part I

Orientation Principles

Chapter 1

The Rationale for Orientation

HISTORY OF ORIENTATION

Orientation programs are a recent development in hospitals. For most of its history, orientation consisted of one person showing another person what to do. Unfortunately, many people did not receive even that simple introduction to a new job. Assuming that anyone hired for a job should already know what to do, many supervisors merely led a new employee to the unit, said "You will work here," and disappeared. The employee was left to flounder alone.

Until the 1930s a hospital worker was a nurse. There might have been a few spare groundskeepers around, and here and there someone to stoke the boiler, but almost everything else was done by nurses, from patient care to cleaning to preparing food. It's not very surprising that the first organized orientation programs were for nurses. When hospitals had their own training programs, instructors usually also served as hospital supervisors. Somewhere along the line someone realized that a nurse who was not trained at that particular hospital needed to learn about the ways that institution differed from the nurse's previous one, and orientation was born.

The growth of orientation programs was accelerated, as were so many other things in health care, by World War II. Suddenly nurses were mobile. Rather than training in a hospital and working there until marriage or retirement ended employment, a nurse could travel all over the country as an officer in the armed services. That wanderlust has never left the profession—a certain percentage of every hospital's turnover represents nurses who just want to move on.

The changes in the nursing profession were accompanied by profound changes in health care as an industry. A technological explosion began that has continued to this day. In the early part of the century one could leave hospital work and return 20 years later to pick up practically where one had left off. Patient care was patient care. After the war, change became the main constant in health care. At present a worker's knowledge and skills may be outdated after only two years away from the hospital; soon the period will be even shorter. Orientation programs are a way of providing the knowledge of new breakthroughs and of updating skills of workers who have been away.

Another change in health care relates to the proliferation of new categories of workers. Since almost the entire staff in hospitals before World War II consisted of nurses, when nurses went to war they left a huge gap in the hospital work force. This gap was filled with unskilled workers trained by the hospitals to give patient care. Nurse attendants, orderlies, and practical nurses soon became not just a stopgap measure but a continuing and necessary component of hospital personnel. As technological advances escalated, new categories were developed for workers who operated the increasingly sophisticated machines that became more and more a part of the industry. Respiratory therapists, ECG technicians, radiology technicians, physical therapists, laboratory technicians—the list of new health care categories is still growing as advances in the health sciences continue.

All of these workers need to be oriented to their jobs and to the institutions for which they work. For years the only education conducted within hospital systems was for nurses ("Nursing Inservice"—the old title is still visible in some hospitals). The new trend is toward hospitalwide education departments involved in the orientation and continuing education of all categories of workers. Future instructors will be responsible for orienting not only nurses but also technicians, laundry workers, accounting personnel, maintenance workers, security officers—the entire gamut of employees.

COSTS OF ORIENTATION

How much does it cost to orient new employees? Most figures are for nurses. A 1976 study (using data from 1973-74) found that orientation costs for 5,865 hospitals totaled $76 million.[1] That figure represented only direct salary costs, ignoring such expenses as fringe benefits and indirect costs of classes. A new RN in the study sample received between 84 and 154 hours of orientation at a salary cost (orientee plus instructors) of between $770 and $984 per orientee.[2]

A more recent study of costs from a single hospital reported a total of 240 hours of general orientation, including classroom and clinical hours. Not including fringe benefits, indirect costs, or instructor time, the direct cost per nurse was $1,512.[3]

Huntington Memorial Hospital in Pasadena, California, has been doing a cost analysis of orientation classes showing both the cost per learner hour and the total cost (including salary) for orienting hospital personnel. In Table 1–1 these figures are broken down by various category of worker. Notice that the amounts relate only to orientation classes. If you include the salary paid to a new worker in the nonproductive period of becoming familiar with the job, the cost skyrockets. Another important relationship illustrated in Table 1–1 is that the cost per learner hour falls as the number of learners in the class rises. This implies that it is more cost effective to have larger orientation classes, an issue that will be discussed again in Chapter 4.

The current problems of rising expenses and falling revenues are causing hospital administrators to take a long, hard look at the expense columns of the budget. Education is often one of the first items to be slashed during an economy drive, and the high costs of orientation make it an especially tempting target. What benefits can be cited to justify spending large amounts of money on orientation?

Table 1–1 Cost Analysis Data on Orientation Classes

New Employee Orientation (one day) (Mixed group of participants, including general employees and nursing personnel)	
Total labor expense (instructors):	$210.56
Total material/fee costs:	118.44
Total hour expense—learner: (47 learners × 6 contact hours × hourly rate)	2501.34
Cost per learner:	60.22
Cost per learner hour:	10.04
Nursing Orientation (four days) (4 RNs, 2 LVNs, 4 NAs)	
Total labor expense (instructors):	633.25
Total material/fee costs:	212.80
Total hour expense—learner:	2089.11
Cost per learner:	277.59
Cost per learner hour:	20.96
New Graduate Orientation (four seminars) (42 new graduate nurses—these seminars *in addition* to regular nursing orientation)	
Total labor expense (instructors):	644.67
Total material/fee costs:	63.50
Total hour expense—learner:	14,085.12
Cost per learner:	352.22
Cost per learner hour:	11.00

Source: Joyce Johnson, Director of Education, Huntington Memorial Hospital, Pasadena, California. Reprinted with permission.

BENEFITS OF ORIENTATION

For the Orientee

Any person entering a new environment for the first time feels uncertain and a little fearful. The job arena can be particularly threatening, not only because one needs a steady income to feel secure but also because our society often defines a person through the job performed. There is tremendous pressure to "prove" oneself when starting a new job. Most people also have a great desire to fit in with their new work group and become accepted members.

A formal orientation process can help ease these burdens for the new employee in several ways. First, orientation classes provide a relatively nonthreatening environment for new people, a chance to "catch their breath" and begin to learn the system. Second, the classes can give orientees valuable information about the institution—philosophy, policies and procedures, forms, equipment, mores, and standards. With this introduction new employees begin to get a feel for the hospital before having to face their peers and demonstrate competence. For example, knowing the intricacies of the hospital's charting system gives confidence to new nurses, enabling them to concentrate on learning their roles rather than on where to record the blood pressure.

Perhaps the biggest benefit of orientation for new employees is the gradual socialization it allows. Moving into a new role is always difficult, and the orientee must adjust to many roles: *new employee* of this unfamiliar organization with its different ways of doing things, strange rules, and new equipment; *new worker* in the individual department with its own folkways, standards, and expectations; and, perhaps most threatening of all, *new individual* in the peer group. Will co-workers be supportive, indifferent, or actively hostile? Will they ever become friends? Facing the myriad uncertainties of being new can be traumatic. In the privileged position of "orientee" the employee can become familiar with the expectations of new roles without having to immediately become productive.

For the Organization

The orientation process also benefits the hospital, an important point to keep in mind when justifying the cost. New employees unfamiliar with correct policies and procedures can be a legal liability, especially in patient care areas. Mistakes and safety hazards can entail expensive corrections and even possible lawsuits. If an employee is injured on the job, costs can be astronomical. Information on safety presented in new employee orientation prevents mishaps. Explaining what equipment is used in the hospital and how it should be operated prevents costly breakdowns and improves patient safety, whether the equipment is an infusion pump, a boiler, a copying machine, or a CAT scanner.

An often overlooked benefit of orientation is the infusion of loyalty it can provide. Society has changed drastically, and managers can no longer expect to merely give directions and be obeyed. Workers are questioning authority, asking the rationale for changes and instructions. When so much is dependent on willing cooperation, on encouraging employees to work *with* the hospital rather than for (or even against) it, loyalty to the organization is priceless. The only way to foster such a feeling is to show employees that the hospital honestly cares about them and their needs.

The very concept of orientation—providing a protected environment in which key information is given—shows concern for the individual and his or her adjustment to the organization. Providing this simple transition gets the message across loud and clear: we care. We want to help so that you can become a productive member of our health care team. Information such as the history of the hospital, how it is organized, the names of the administrators and other key people, helps the new employee identify with the organization and its goals. This initial identification will pay off later in higher productivity, fewer mistakes, and a decreased turnover rate.

EFFECTS OF ORIENTATION ON EMPLOYEES

Surprisingly little research has been done on the effects of orientation on the adjustment of the employee to the organization. One interesting study investigated exactly what happens to a person who begins working in a hospital. Dr. Daniel Charles Feldman of Northwestern University's Graduate School of Management examined the organizational socialization of hospital employees—"a study of the ways employees are transformed from total outsiders of organizations to participating and effective members of them."[4] He discovered three distinct stages of the socialization process, each with its own set of indicators for judging how smoothly the process is going.

Stages of Organizational Socialization

Stage One: Anticipatory Socialization encompasses all learning that occurs before the person enters the organization. The indicators are *realism,* the extent to which the individual has a full and accurate picture of what life in the organization is really like, and *congruence,* the extent to which the person and the organization "fit" together and meet each other's needs.

Stage Two: Accommodation is the period in which the individual sees what the organization is really like and attempts to become a member of it. The indicators are *initiation to the task,* the extent to which an employee feels competent to perform the job; *initiation to the group,* the extent to which an employee feels accepted and trusted by co-workers; *role definition,* an agreement with the work group on what tasks to perform and how they should be prioritized; and *congruence of evaluation,* the extent to which an employee and supervisor similarly evaluate the employee's progress within the organization.

Stage Three: Role Management involves mediation of conflicts between work life and home life and conflicts between the employee's work group and other groups in the organization. The indicators are *resolution of outside life conflicts* and *resolution of conflicting demands.*[5]

Implications for Orientation

Placing these stages in hospital education terms, we can see that anticipatory socialization corresponds with the recruitment phase of employment. In most institutions the people responsible for orientation have no input or influence in this phase. They merely receive a list of names of the people beginning work and their dates of hire. However, the importance of an honest description of both the pros and cons of the job during the hiring interview should be obvious.

Accommodation is the stage in which orientation takes place. The impact of formal classes and clinical experience to help new employees adjust to their roles cannot be overemphasized. Without an orderly transition from outsider to employee, the initiation to tasks and group will be rocky, role definition unclear, and the likelihood of employee and supervisor feeling the same way about end-of-probation performance uncertain.

At first glance orientation would seem to have little to do with the third stage of socialization, which generally takes place between the end of the third month and the end of the first year of employment.[6] The long-term impact of a thorough orientation is still controversial, but a number of hospitals have noted dramatic drops in turnover rates and an increase in statements of satisfaction from new employees when a formal orientation program is adopted.[7]

CONCLUSION

Hospital orientation developed as a result of the myriad social pressures resulting from World War II, which caused tremendous changes in the health care field. The increasing costs of orienting new employees must be weighed against the many benefits identified by both workers and organizations. The process of orientation can have a dramatic impact on socialization of new employees, increasing satisfaction and adjustment to the new role, and decreasing turnover.

The next chapter will examine what content should be included in orientation, how to assess employee needs, and how to use those assessment results in planning orientation.

NOTES

1. S.H. Kase and B. Swenson, *Costs of Hospital-Sponsored Orientation and Inservice Education for Registered Nurses* (Bethesda, Md.: DHEW Publication No. (HRA) 77-25, U.S. Department of Health, Education, and Welfare, November 1976): 27–38.

2. Ibid., 38.

3. Margaret D. Sovie, "The Role of Staff Development in Hospital Cost Control," *Journal of Nursing Administration* 10, no. 11 (November 1980): 39.

4. Daniel Charles Feldman, "Organizational Socialization of Hospital Employees," *Medical Care* 15, no. 10 (October 1977): 799.

5. Ibid., 800–801.

6. Ibid., 806.

7. *Analyzing and Reducing Employee Turnover in Hospitals* (New York: United Hospital Fund of New York, 1968), 49–52; and Christine Fredericks, "Reversing the Turnover Trend," *Nursing Management* 12, no. 12 (December 1981): 42–44.

SUGGESTED READINGS

Deloughery, Grace L. *History and Trends of Professional Nursing*, 8th ed. St. Louis: C.V. Mosby Co., 1977.

DeYoung, Lillian. *Dynamics of Nursing*, 4th ed. St. Louis: C.V. Mosby Co., 1981.

Heiderken, L. "Inservice Education and Research." *Nursing Outlook* 7 (1959).

McNally, Jean. *Continuing Education for Nurses*. Kansas City: American Nurses Association, 1972.

Miller, M.A. "Trends of Inservice Education." In *The Yearbook of Professional Nursing*, edited by C. Cowan. New York: G.P. Putnam's Sons, 1956.

Pfefferkorn, B. "Improvement of the Nurse in Service—An Historical Review." *American Journal of Nursing* 28 (1928).

Poole, D. "Inservice Education Reaches a Milestone." *American Journal of Nursing* 53 (1953).

Rowland, Howard S., ed. *The Nurse's Almanac*. Rockville, Md.: Aspen Systems Corporation, 1978.

Tobin, Helen M., and Judy S. Wengerd. "What Makes a Staff Development Program Work?" *American Journal of Nursing* 71 (1971).

Chapter 2
Selection of Content

What should be taught in orientation? The information that could be presented seems overwhelming. Policies, procedures, employee benefits—once you start listing important things to cover you realize that orientation fits comfortably into a month of eight-hour class days. However, no hospital could afford that much class time and no employee could stand to spend that much time sitting in class.

Only certain vital information can be covered in the limited time available. How do you decide what to include? One way *not* to do it is to follow tradition. With change the only constant in the health care environment, "We've always done it that way" is a signal to take a long, hard look at the content.

Everything taught in orientation must contribute to the overall goal of the program: providing new employees with the information needed to become productive, satisfied members of the hospital team. To accomplish this, everyone with a stake in new employees' success should participate in the orientation process.

DECISION MAKERS

Who should be involved in choosing the information to be covered in orientation? Whatever you do, don't try to decide by yourself. Not only will your judgments about what is currently happening in the clinical areas be faulty, you will definitely need the support of line personnel. Managers and staff are vital to the ultimate success of any orientation program. Enlisting their help not only ensures the input of relevant information for the classes, it will automatically elicit support and interest for the whole endeavor.

Managers

The hospital managers are the first people to approach. Talk to the chief administrator: how does he or she perceive the orientation program? Is it seen as effective . . . current . . . a total waste of time and money? What information would the administrator like to see included in orientation? This executive has valuable input because he or she sees the "big picture"—the hospital as an organizational entity with economic and sociopolitical ties to the community and the nation. Knowing the long-term goals of the organization, the outside influences impacting on its needs and services, the chief executive officer is an invaluable source of information on orientation content.

An interview also provides an opportunity to inform this all-important allocator of resources about your program and its contribution to patient care. During your meeting, explain that authorities feel that job satisfaction begins in the initial orientation period.[1] The more effectively the orientation period can contribute to retention of staff and increased productivity, the better off the hospital will be. With the administrator's help, you intend to make the program the best it can be.

Repeat this interview with the assistant administrators: what are their ideas about orientation? Some will have few suggestions, but your main purpose will have been achieved. The decision makers of the hospital will be aware of the orientation program and will remember that you asked for their input.

At the department head and head nurse level questioning should become more specific. What problems have occurred with orientees? Could any of them have been prevented by more comprehensive orientation classes? At this point you have to focus attention on what can realistically be presented in an orientation program. Preparing a new employee to function comfortably in a new environment does not include skills training in every nursing procedure that should have been practiced in school. Nor does making the new person feel a part of the organization mean that every department in the hospital should present what they do and how they do it. One of the most common problems of orientation programs is information overload.[2] Be sure the managers understand that you are gathering all the ideas and suggestions you can but that not everything can or will be included in the classes.

This is especially important at the first-line supervisor level (assistant head nurses, team leaders, allied department supervisors). These front-line managers will have both the most valuable suggestions and the most impossible demands. "Why don't you teach the orientees how to be in charge?" "Be sure they know where all the equipment is kept before they come on the unit." How can you reconcile these demands with the limited time available? You can't. Without refusing to include any specific suggestion (remember, you want to encourage their input), make it clear that orientees will be responsible for learning many of the details after classes are completed. And the first-line supervisors are the ones who will be seen as resource people during this period. Let them know that and solicit their support.

As you can tell, the process of gathering information from the managers is also a recruiting effort. Use the interview as a way to build rapport with these crucial people so that they perceive you as an ally in the business of hiring and retaining new employees. Set appointments and keep them—they may be late, you should not. Take detailed notes of their comments and suggestions, and ask questions to be sure you understand exactly what the managers see as the problems and solutions. Show interest and enthusiasm for the program. You want the hospital to support orientation, so demonstrate that you feel it is not only important but vital to improving productivity and lessening turnover.

Employees

Nonmanagement personnel have valuable ideas about orientation and how to improve it. Employees work with new people, answer their questions, observe the adjustment problems they have. They are also the ones who have to cope with the difficulties that arise when new employees operate with incomplete, incorrect, or misunderstood information. To tap into this well of ideas, talk to the staff. You can't interview every employee in the hospital, but speak to a representative sampling—at least one person from every department.

Employees who have recently been orientees themselves are your single most valuable source of information. How did they feel during orientation? Did the classes help them adjust to their new environment? Was too much covered? If so, what should be eliminated? What helped the most? The least? Could anything have been presented in a different format for better retention? What are their suggestions for scheduling classes? Did they feel that their individual needs were considered and addressed?

Besides one-to-one interviews, some hospitals are now conducting three-month meetings with new employees. The department head or division director meets formally with a group of new personnel after the probationary period to get feedback on the orientation process and the orientees' adjustment to the hospital. Ask that all pertinent information from this meeting be sent to you.

Orientees

A frequently overlooked source of information on what should be taught during orientation is the orientee. Too often we get locked into teaching content with the philosophy "They need to know this, so I'm going to teach it." But is there a better way for new employees to learn this all-important information? Or do they know it already? The only way to find out is to ask. Orientees at many hospitals now identify their own learning needs right at the start of orientation through knowledge and skill inventories.[3]

If you're dealing with two to five people in a group, begin your part of their orientation with an interview. What is their background and experience? Have they worked with primary care? What sort of charting and care plans are they used

Exhibit 2–1 Learning Styles Questionnaire

Learning Styles Self-Assessment

1. Describe how you learn best—lecture, self-study, role-playing, demonstration, etc.
2. Describe your greatest asset in terms of learning.
3. Describe your greatest limitation in terms of learning.
4. If it could be perfect, what would you get out of this orientation?

to? With a large group this may have to be done by questionnaire or by going around the room with each person giving a brief summary of past experience.

The most important thing to discover about the orientees is how they learn. Individual learning styles can impact dramatically on retention of content, as will be discussed in Chapter 4. Exhibit 2–1 is an example of a questionnaire used to elicit information about learning styles from orientees. Using such a guide, an instructor can alter the approach to the material. For instance, if you discover the group learns better by participation, use more charting exercises and case studies and decrease the lecture time. Orientee input can actually alter your teaching strategies.

Education Department Instructors

The professional educators of the hospital are responsible for taking a mass of data and molding it into a manageable curriculum. You are the expert on delivery of orientation—how the learners will best absorb and retain the information they need to function in the hospital system. Using the facts and feelings collected from the rest of the organization, you will have to decide what should be included in the classes and what should wait until the orientees reach a later point in the process.

One source that cannot be ignored is the Joint Commission on Accreditation of Hospitals (JCAH). This organization has set standards for orientation content that must be included and documented if the hospital is to remain accredited. For instance, these are the orientation guidelines for the dietary department:

> New personnel shall receive an orientation of sufficient duration and substance prior to providing dietetic services without direct supervision. This orientation shall be documented. As appropriate to their level of responsibility, such individuals shall receive instruction and demonstrate competence in:

- Personal hygiene and infection control
- The proper inspection, handling, preparation, serving, and storing of food
- The proper cleaning and safe operation of equipment
- General foodservice sanitation and safety
- The proper method of waste disposal
- Portion control
- The writing of modified diets using the diet manual/handbook
- Diet instruction
- The recording of pertinent dietetic information in the patient's medical record.[4]

This is only an excerpt from a single department's guidelines! If you have not already done so, read the JCAH manual from cover to cover, underlining in red all parts that pertain to orientation, and marking those pages with paper clips for easy reference.

One way to base content decisions on facts rather than feelings is to conduct a formal needs assessment. The more information you have about the hospital system and what successful employees need to know, the more defensible your choice of class content will be.

NEEDS ASSESSMENT IN THE HOSPITAL

Knowles defines a learning need as "something a person ought to learn for his own good, for the good of an organization, or for the good of society."[5] A needs assessment can be conducted through a variety of methods, but the educator must keep firmly in mind the caveat that the good of the organization includes controlling the expense of the assessment process. Table 2–1 lists possible methods of needs assessment with their advantages and disadvantages. As each is discussed, think of how these methods could be applied to your own situation.

Direct Observation

Tobin, Yoder-Wise, and Hull feel that direct observation of work performance is probably the best method of identifying needs.[6] To help future orientees, watch how the present ones perform. What problems can be seen in the care they give, the tasks they do? Do the problems stem from learning needs: is a lack of knowledge causing them to perform incorrectly? Or are the orientees having problems because there are organizational barriers to good performance? If new people are not encouraged to do things right, if they don't receive help and support

Table 2–1 Methods of Learning Needs Assessment in the Hospital

Method	*Advantages*	*Disadvantages*
Direct observation	Can see application of learning. Immediate data. Instructor visibility. Available to help orientees.	Time consuming. May be seen as "spy." Subjective. Difficult to gather adequate sampling.
Interviews	Direct contact with decision makers. Able to explore answers. Gives people a feeling of ownership in the program. Easy to direct and keep on target.	Time consuming. Interviewer may affect responses. Difficult to gather adequate sampling. Interviewees may expect all data to be used.
Records and reports	Easily accessible. Provide clues to overall hospital functioning. May be analyzed for patterns.	Time consuming. Data may be hard to interpret. May indicate organizational problems rather than learning needs.
Job analysis and performance review	Specific, precise information gathered about job categories. Represent actual on-the-job performance. Easy to analyze job tasks that must be taught.	Time consuming. May not be current. Confidentiality of employees must be maintained.
Surveys	Provide broad sampling of employee opinion. Usually easy to compose and administer.	May be superficial, unvalidated information. Much of the data may be inapplicable.
Advisory committees and other committees	Provide input from many departments. Members familiar with the needs of their areas.	Membership may not be representative. Assignment and purpose may be unclear.
Skills inventories	Individualize needs assessment. Provide for orientee input. Quick and easy to administer.	Often too long and detailed. May be inaccurately completed.
Tests	Quickly identify deficiencies. Results easy to compile and report. Objective comparison of orientees.	Must be validated. Give clues but not conclusive.

from the line personnel who work with them, changing the content of orientation is not likely to help.

It is very important that observations be done systematically, to ensure a full sampling of all areas and shifts. It may help to prepare an observation tool to help gather information. As the observations progress it will become easier to spot key performance factors. If it seems that there is just too much to see and take note of, try observing a single facet of performance. For example, Exhibit 2–2 shows the observations of a nurse passing medications. Notice how problems are exposed—not just time management problems on the nurse's part but, even more strongly, problems with the system of care delivery.

Because you may uncover a number of problems, be sure to let managers and staff know what you are doing and why. Enlist their help at the beginning so that you won't be perceived as a spy come to find mistakes and get them into trouble.

Interviews

The process of interviewing managers and staff has been discussed in the section on decision makers but one group that has a wealth of data about employee

---

Exhibit 2–2 Observations of Medication Nurse

8:40 Took pain pill to pt. + brought 9 o'clocks with it. No water at bedside. Went to kitchen, filled water pitcher, back to rm., helped pt. take meds. Also brought water for other pt.

8:47 Checked med. book with Kardex. Answered 2 NAs questions.

9:00 Put sheets with new orders in book. Checked syringe + needle supply on cart; restocked. Attached paper sack for trash to cart.

9:04 Called by NA to talk to pt. over intercom—question for nurse. Placed note for Dr. on chart.

9:07 Began passing meds. 724 just back from x-ray, wanted coffee. Passed request to NA.

9:10 Pt. handed nurse STAT urine specimen. Took to station, ran order, attached sticker, gave to NA.

9:13 Talked to "special" in 727—meds. already given. Had special initial the book.

9:14 728—medicine (B_{12} and B complex) not in cassette. Made out back-up slip and gave rest of meds. Had to put bed up + explain to pt. (slightly confused). Took each pill very slowly. Put bed back down.

9:19 Special from 727 needed pain pill. Team leader went to station, unlocked narcotic drawer, gave it to nurse, charged it, put it in narcotics book.

9:21 729—Reconstituted Methicillin dose. Pt. refused meds. until she got her eye gtts.—not in cassette. Found in bedside table. Instilled while still trying to get Methicillin dissolved. Gave in divided doses. Noted irritated area on body—looked like tape allergy. Talked to pt. about it.

9:35 730—Poured + mixed 3 regular meds. Added Neosporin to GU irrigant. Pt. crying but couldn't say why. Explored with pt., finally ascertained that she was in pain. Went to station for PRN med. Crushed tablet with mortar + pestle, mixed with custard (had to go to kitchen). Gave all meds. to pt. very slowly to avoid choking. Pt. clutching nurse's hand, wouldn't let go. Moaned and cried. Nurse soothed her. Recorded I+O.

Now 9:48 A.M.—nurse has 12 more patients to administer medications to and chart the results of these rounds.

performance has yet to be explored. Through patient interviews you can discover if the information taught in orientation is being applied to patient care.

Whether you're interviewing clients about nursing care, food service, housekeeping services, or the care given by any department, from the business office to radiology, decide what information you want and develop questions to probe for it. One of the advantages of interviewing is that the facts are fresh in the patient's mind. Establish that you need this data to help you improve care for everyone, and most clients participate willingly. Involving family members provides fresh insights, since they perceive the care given from yet another angle.

It may be wise to promise anonymity, as some people are afraid that a negative comment might cause repercussions from the nursing staff. It would be nice to think that such a thing is impossible, but probably better for the patient's peace of mind to keep names and room numbers out of the reports of these interviews.

Records and Reports

The burgeoning quantities of paperwork involved in health care can provide valuable information for hospital educators. No matter what department is being studied, somewhere there is a record or report providing data on its functioning that will shed light on learning needs.

Patient Questionnaires

The percentage of patient questionnaires returned is usually quite small, but when a questionnaire is sent back it often means the client felt strongly about some aspect of his or her care. Note both the positive and negative feedback, since you need to know what the organization is doing right, as well as identify problems.

Incident Reports

Analysis of the mistakes and accidents from all areas underlines problems to emphasize to new employees. A number of medications given incorrectly may indicate weakness in the administration system or an epidemic of carelessness. If you study individual reports, a pattern should emerge. Perhaps employees are not checking patient identification, or physicians' orders are being transcribed incorrectly. Based on this information you can stress the needed safeguards during orientation. The same process can be used to analyze patient falls, infection rates, equipment malfunctions, or any of the problems recorded on these reports.

Nursing Audit

If you are not already on the audit committee, try to arrange for membership at once. Every activity will offer insight into patient care problems. Deficiencies identified by audit require a response from the education department, either through classes or one-on-one instruction on the units; the same information also identifies areas of orientation that should be redefined or emphasized.

Statistical Records

Valuable data can be gleaned from records of turnover, maintenance requests, employee applications, absentee reports, department monthly reports, financial records, and the annual report published by the hospital. To analyze such records efficiently, keep in mind the types of information that you need and target your search. Focus on the variances and discrepancies that have implications for orientation.

The Chart

The record that is at once most helpful and most frustrating is the official patient chart. It is most helpful because reading through the record of the patient's stay identifies more learning needs per hour of effort than almost any other source (except perhaps the staff interview). The frustration comes from the magnitude of the task. Chart analysis is time consuming, sometimes tedious, often confusing. When you supplement reviewing the chart with patient observation and staff interview, a fuller picture of patient care will emerge. Report any errors you discover to the head nurse (yes, you will find some). If the patient care plan is not part of the official record, start a campaign to make it so; prizing care plans enough to make them legal documents is the only way to ensure their completion and maintenance.

Which of the available records and reports you use depends on the information needed. Their accessibility and abundance make them an invaluable asset. But remember that this very accessibility can be a trap—data collection can become an end unto itself. A good rule of thumb might be to limit the time spent analyzing records to no more than 10 percent of the total time of your assessment.

Job Analysis and Performance Review

Many hospitals have linked the process of breaking down jobs into their component tasks and analyzing the skills needed to perform those tasks with the process of performance appraisal. Reviewing the tasks necessary to successfully perform a job, and managers' evaluations of how well those tasks are performed, can yield useful information about learning deficiencies. As you analyze the data, patterns of needs emerge that can be used in planning orientation. Remember that evaluations are confidential documents and protect employee privacy by having names and departments obscured on the copies sent to you.

Surveys

The easiest way to get opinions on learning needs from a large number of employees is through a survey. When designing the questionnaire to be used, remember that multiple-choice check-off answers (see Exhibit 2–3) make it easier to compile results but limit the amount of information you receive. Open-ended questions (see Exhibit 2–4) garner more responses but make it difficult to organize the results. Whether you use check-off or open-ended questions, keep in mind that much of the data you collect may not prove helpful in planning class content, since the respondents may be unclear about the purpose of the survey, may have felt it was not important, and are expressing subjective opinions that you cannot explore in more depth.

Committees

Representatives of various departments meet periodically to advise hospital educators on needs in their areas. Membership may be limited to managers, or include some workers as well. An advisory committee serves as a sounding board for the education department. A well-functioning committee can offer information, support, and follow-up provided by no other entity in the organization. The keys to an effective advisory body are (1) intelligent, well-thought-out selection of members and (2) strong guidance toward a clearly defined purpose. Since both of these are the responsibility of the educators, the blame for a poorly functioning committee rests squarely on their shoulders.

Other committees can also contribute to orientation efforts. The policy and procedures committee composes and updates the guidelines for hospital practice. Disaster is guaranteed if the orientation instructors aren't informed of changes or new policies and procedures. The best way to keep informed is to be on the committee. If that proves impossible, be sure all minutes are routed to you. Identify other committees that are sources of learning needs—pharmacy committee, care planning committee, cardiac arrest committee, etc.—and keep the lines of communication open.

Skills Inventories

Lists of skills or tasks needed to perform a job adequately can be compiled and given to orientees to rank their own abilities. Usually the ranking is divided into such categories as "Experienced," "Need supervision," or "Need instruction" (see Exhibit 2–5). Getting a needs assessment from orientees ensures personalization of at least part of the orientation process, if the information is used. If it won't be used, don't gather it. Avoid skills inventories the length of the New York

Exhibit 2–3 Education Questionnaire for RNs and LVNs

Topic	*Very interested*	*Interested*	*Not interested*
Law and the Nurse	_____	_____	_____
Handling Sudden Condition Changes	_____	_____	_____
Documenting Patient Care	_____	_____	_____
Update in Pharmacology	_____	_____	_____
Infection Control and the Nurse	_____	_____	_____
Sexuality: Implications for Patient Care	_____	_____	_____
The Nurse's Role in a Disaster	_____	_____	_____
Nursing Audit and Standards of Care	_____	_____	_____

Please list other topics you would like covered:

	Very interested	Interested
____________________	_______	_______
____________________	_______	_______
____________________	_______	_______
____________________	_______	_______

Please list the days of the week and times of day most convenient:

	Day(s) of week	Time(s) of day
Full-day workshop	_________	_________
Half-day workshop	_________	_________
One-hour workshop	_________	_________

Source: Education Department, Huntington Memorial Hospital, Pasadena, California. Reprinted with permission.

telephone directory—anything longer than three pages is unwieldy and the orientees will probably not devote enough time to completing it. Another problem with skills inventories develops when an orientee feels uncomfortable admitting that certain skills need improvement. If the inventory is completed inaccurately, it will be hard to provide needed experience. Validate all inventory results with on-the-job observation.

Exhibit 2–4 Open-ended Education Questionnaire

Education Needs Survey for 1983

Part I: Please list the subjects you would like to have presented to you and your staff which would assist you in maintaining or upgrading your own or your department's performance.

	Subject	Priority #
1.		
2.		
3.		
4.		
5.		

Part II: Prioritize the above five subjects in the second column with the most crucial need as #1.

Part III: If you would like to present a program yourself, but need assistance in developing the content or structuring the class, please indicate the topic and the projected date of presentation and we will try to provide the assistance you require.

	Subject	Projected date
1.		
2.		

Submitted by ______________________ Date ______________
Department ______________________ Ext. ______________

Thank you for your time in filling out this form. If you have any questions feel free to call the Education Department.

Source: Education Department, Huntington Memorial Hospital, Pasadena, California. Reprinted with permission.

Tests

Tobin, Yoder-Wise, and Hull list two reasons for using pretests as a basis for identifying learning needs: (1) to determine whether or not individuals have knowledge and skills that are necessary for participation in a specific offering and (2) to determine what participants already know based on the learning objectives of the offering.[7] The hiring interview should ensure that the prerequisite knowledge and skills for orientation are present, but this is not always the case. For example, some nurses lack the knowledge of drugs and their effects that a hospital feels is necessary for safe patient care. The only way to assess the level of drug knowledge of all orientees *before* they reach the patients is through testing. If such a test is administered prior to hiring it must be validated.

Exhibit 2–5 Nursing Skills Inventory

New Nurse Experience Checklist

Procedure	*No experience*	*Would like supervision*	*Confident*
Enemas	______	______	______
Catheterization	______	______	______
Tracheal suction	______	______	______
Tracheostomy care	______	______	______
Complete isolation	______	______	______
Ostomy care	______	______	______
Starting IVs	______	______	______
IV Medications	______	______	______
Insertion of NG tubes	______	______	______
Care of pt./chest tubes	______	______	______
Care of pt. in traction	______	______	______
Sterile irrigations	______	______	______
Abdominal wound care	______	______	______
Decubitus care	______	______	______
Team leading	______	______	______
Use of IV infusion pumps	______	______	______
Others:______			

Validity refers to the degree to which a particular device measures what it is intended to measure.[8] A pharmacology test must be validated by administering it to a representative sampling of staff nurses, perhaps one or two from each unit. Ensuring anonymity helps obtain volunteers. Score the tests and do an item analysis, noting how many people missed each question. If a large number of respondents missed an item, it should be revised or deleted. Repeat this process until you have a test that nurses currently giving medications in your facility can pass. That test can now be considered valid for your hospital.

Even with a validated test the hospital can run into legal problems if it is administered as a condition of hire. Applicants can challenge the fairness of the test, or can claim that it discriminates against people of a particular national origin. Certainly you would have to be careful that it was administered in exactly the same way to everyone applying for a position. One way around this dilemma is to give the test *after* hire. The policy might be that a nurse must pass the test before being allowed to administer medications. If the test is failed, the nurse could have the option to study and retake it or to enroll in a pharmacology course. Remember that the goal is to develop knowledgeable, safe practitioners, not to see how difficult you can make the test or how many nurses can be "washed out." Exhibit 2–6 is an excerpt from a test used in one hospital.

Exhibit 2–6 Pharmacology Test

1. Digoxin and digitoxin are:
   a. Two different drugs belonging to the same family
   b. Two different names for the same drug
   c. Drugs closely related enough that they could be substituted for each other
   d. Have no relation to each other
2. When the patient develops urticaria and pruritis following a dose of antibiotic, you would:
   a. Record the observation in the patient's chart
   b. Observe the patient frequently for progression of the reaction
   c. Notify the physician
   d. All of the above
3. The major side effect of long term streptomycin therapy is:
   a. Urticaria
   b. G.I. distress
   c. Damage to the 8th cranial nerve
4. If a patient indicates that as a child he had a reaction to an antibiotic you are giving him, you would:
   a. Tell him it is okay to take the drug; you will be near if he has any problems
   b. Hold the drug and notify the physician
   c. Tell him to take the drug—a childhood reaction has no significance to the present
   d. Skip the dose
5. What substance(s) should not be taken at the same time that streptomycin is taken?
   1. Milk 2. Orange juice 3. Maalox
      a. 1 only
      b. 1 and 3
      c. 2 and 3
      d. All of the above

Determining what orientees already know about the objectives of the offering prevents repeating already-learned information in class. For example, administering a pretest on legal aspects of nursing (Exhibit 2–7) enables participants to demonstrate their knowledge of the subject, saves class time, and leads into discussion of the key points. Tests can be used in many different subjects, from infection control to laundry procedures.

ASSESSMENT RESULTS IN COURSE PLANNING

The more sources of data you tap during your needs assessment, the more reliable your results are likely to be. Although few instructors have the time or budget to use all the methods discussed, be sure to explore more than just interviews or just testing or just observation.

Working with this mass of data is like assembling a huge jigsaw puzzle. The framework goes together easily, but the central parts are difficult to fit into a

Exhibit 2–7 Pretest for Orientation Class

Legal Implications for Nurses

Instructions: Circle the correct answer.

1.	Professional negligence is always a criminal act.	T	F
2.	Nurses can be held liable and successfully sued if their actions, even unintentionally, cause injury to a patient.	T	F
3.	A nurse's failure to act carries less liability than acting improperly, when either causes injury to a patient.	T	F
4.	Nurses have the duty to do everything within their power to ensure patients are protected from malpractice by other professionals, including physicians.	T	F
5.	If an adult patient for any reason cannot sign a consent form, the signature of a spouse or other close relative makes the document legally proper.	T	F
6.	If a physician has not already done so, it is the nurse's responsibility to make clear to the patient sufficient information about proposed surgical procedures (including all risks and hazards), to enable the patient to give an informed consent.	T	F

Source: Education Department, Huntington Memorial Hospital, Pasadena, California. Reprinted with permission.

coherent pattern. One way to organize it is to list the overall goals as the first step. A goal is a broad, general statement denoting the purpose of a training program; it sets the tone for the more specific behavioral objectives to follow.[9] What do you hope to accomplish from the orientation process? What benefits will accrue for the patients? For the hospital? For the orientees? Don't worry about wording—you are organizing your thoughts in order to provide direction and focus for the program.

Once the goals are established, list the major topics that should be treated within each general content area. Depending on what needs your assessment revealed, some major topics might be "Policies," "Charting," "Infection Control." These provide the general basis for instruction. Analyze your findings, eliminating contradictions and data not applicable to orientation. Each time a topic is reinforced from another data source, indicate that it should receive extra emphasis. It quickly becomes clear that some areas are more important than others. Be sure to consider the source: input from managers and staff will have more impact than information from some of the other sources.

Now decide your general purpose for each topic. You are not writing objectives, you are describing broad outcomes. These are your own personal aims and purposes for each segment. Once you are clear about the direction and focus of the orientation program, you will be ready to tackle preparing learning objectives.

CONCLUSION

Interviewing key people and conducting an institutional needs assessment ensures that all pertinent data sources have been tapped. Setting priorities and organizing content into manageable sessions is a formidable task, but working from information specific to the hospital enables you to approach this job with confidence.

Chapter 3 will deal with the next step in planning orientation content: setting objectives for the total program and for individual sessions. These objectives will be the cornerstones for scheduling, teaching, and evaluating orientation.

NOTES

1. M.E.G.A. Beekman, "The Need for Inservice Education for Nursing with Suggestions for Its Organization," *The Lamp* 29, no. 2 (February 1972): 22.

2. Calvin P. Otto and Rollin O. Glaser, *The Management of Training* (Reading, Mass.: Addison-Wesley Publishing Co., 1970), 342.

3. Margaret D. Sovie, "Investigate Before You Educate," *The Journal of Nursing Administration* 11, no. 4 (April 1981): 17.

4. *Accreditation Manual for Hospitals, 1983 Edition* (Chicago: Joint Commission on Accreditation of Hospitals, 1983), 16–17.

5. Malcolm S. Knowles, *The Modern Practice of Adult Education* (Chicago: Association Press, Follett Publishing Co., 1980), 88.

6. Helen M. Tobin, Pat S. Yoder-Wise, and Peggy K. Hull, *The Process of Staff Development: Components for Change*, 3d ed. (St. Louis: C.V. Mosby Co., 1979), 103.

7. Ibid., 108.

8. Jean E. Schweer, *Creative Teaching in Clinical Nursing*, 3d ed. (St. Louis: C.V. Mosby Co., 1976), 169.

9. Corinne B. Linton, "Training," in *Hospital-Based Education*, ed. Corinne B. Linton and James W. Truelove (New York: Arco Publishing, 1980), 72.

Chapter 3

Designing Objectives for Orientation

Objectives accomplish many things in the educational process but the most important reason for having orientation objectives is a practical, organizational one. As we have seen, there is far more content to be covered than any program, no matter how liberal, could accommodate. Orientation programs often become topheavy with "nice-to-know" information and the only remedy for this is careful development of objectives. Otto and Glaser state that "of all hospital education programs, orientation is most likely to get out of hand and is therefore most in need of watching."[1] Armed with information from the needs assessment and your list of overall purposes and topics, use the objective-setting process to control the amount and type of information within the program.

PURPOSES OF OBJECTIVES

Too often, objectives are like classics in literature—everyone says how important they are but few actually read them. How many times has an instructor, pressed for time and not really believing that objectives make much difference, written the class content, selected teaching strategies, chosen evaluation methods, and then scribbled some objectives? Unless instructors realize the value of carefully prepared objectives, they are unlikely to spend much time and thought on them. And if the program objectives are poorly thought out and hastily written, why should participants read them? The whole process becomes a waste of time, and instructors and students lose a valuable tool for understanding and communication.

Broadwell put it forcefully: "The most important single consideration in the teaching-learning process is the setting of objectives. Taken in proper perspective, the entire course, from beginning to end, should revolve around objectives."[2]

What do written objectives accomplish?

1. The process of writing exactly what you expect orientees to be able to do when they finish the program forces a reappraisal of what information should be presented.
2. By reviewing the objectives, instructors can choose teaching strategies based on required behaviors. If the orientee must be able to *state* something, lecture or reading would be appropriate. If the objectives require the orientee to *complete* a care plan, then that activity should be provided through simulation.
3. Objectives help instructors focus on key points in presentations—areas of emphasis are automatically clear.
4. By keying objectives to on-the-job performance, orientation content will maintain relevance and credibility for both orientees and hospital staff.
5. Communicating to new employees exactly what will be expected of them by the end of the program helps them direct their efforts toward accomplishment of targeted outcomes.
6. Clearly stated objectives are invaluable as guidelines for evaluating both the orientees and the orientation process. Did the person accomplish what was expected in the time allotted? If not, what went wrong? By tracking back along the specific objective(s) that were not completed, you can identify if the problem involved the participant, program content, or on-the-job follow-up and reinforcement.

These benefits only accrue if objectives are carefully thought out and clearly written and communicated. It is hard to write realistic objectives because you are trying to predict exactly what orientees will learn from your program. But if you can't state what the orientees will be able to do when they leave your hands, how can you effectively teach them?

DEVELOPING OBJECTIVES

Some experts feel that it is the responsibility of management to provide an instructor with objectives to be achieved in a course.[3] This seems unrealistic for two reasons. First, most managers have neither the time nor the inclination to do this, and without some background in education it would be difficult for a manager to state objectives in any usable form. Second, instructional objectives should be written by the person (or persons) responsible for presenting the material to be learned. The process of writing out the things participants are to achieve is an integral part of developing a course. Without disciplined analysis, the instructor is likely to lose the focus of the program. The result is a diluted potpourri of information presented in no particular order or emphasis.

Should Objectives Be Behavioral?

Anyone who has taken an education course or read any literature in the field has run across the term "behavioral" objectives. When psychologist B.F. Skinner investigated Pavlov's animal experiments, he found that some of them could be replicated with humans and had educational implications. Skinner and other behaviorists researched the responses that humans learned to make in the presence of stimuli and tried to discover rules governing the stimulus-response (S-R) relationship.

Educational psychologists reached eagerly for such a clear-cut approach to education, and for a time the vogue was to teach everything based on the S-R approach. Unfortunately, this proved too simplistic a method for teaching complex courses, and human variables repeatedly affected the outcomes. Although behaviorists' findings have considerable merit, particularly in the area of reinforcement and shaping behavior, the focus in education moved on to new theories.

The greatest benefit derived from the behaviorists' findings was a different approach to writing objectives. Before that time objectives tended to focus on the teacher's activities, not the learners'. Objectives would be stated as, for example, "Encourage an appreciation of music," a totally unmeasurable goal. Using the S-R approach, attention was turned to the *students'* learning—particularly the behaviors they should exhibit in response to the stimuli encountered in class. This proved to be so much clearer and easier to evaluate that behavioral objectives have become widely adopted, although they are now usually called "instructional" or "performance" objectives.

Writing Objectives

Training and Continuing Education: A Handbook for Health Care Institutions states that "Learning is concerned with observable behavior which is to be evaluated with reference to criteria that state how employees are expected to perform. Objectives should describe just what the instructor or evaluator should be able to observe in the employee's performance when the objective has been reached."[4]

Mager states that "An objective is a description of a performance you want learners to be able to exhibit before you consider them competent."[5] In both examples, notice the emphasis on *doing*. When you write objectives you are describing the performance of the participants, not the performance of the instructor. Write objectives with action verbs that state what participants must do to show achievement. If you keep this in mind you will avoid the most common mistake made when writing objectives: listing what the student will learn. "The orientee will learn how to write nursing care plans." "The orientee will understand the organization of the hospital." "The orientee will develop an appreciation of the role of different departments in patient care."

The above objectives are real ones that were actually used in a program. While they may be worthwhile goals, there is no way to tell if they have been achieved, no way to *measure* them. How can I observe someone in the process of "understanding"? Unless I have extraordinary powers of telepathy, I can't. However, I can observe an orientee *writing* care plans, or *sketching* an organization chart, or *listing* the responsibilities that each department has toward patient care.

Levels of Objectives

When writing objectives, the instructor must always keep in mind that measurable objectives are precise statements describing what orientees will be able to do at the end of orientation. To make the task of writing such exact descriptions easier, think of orientation as having two levels: the overall program level and the individual class level. Kemp feels that the first level requires *terminal* objectives, which state what the orientees will do at the end of the program. When points or concepts within the total program are addressed, *interim* or *enabling* objectives are written.[6]

Exhibit 3–1 is an excerpt from the terminal objectives for a nursing orientation program. Notice that each objective describes an action demonstrated by the orientee that either the instructor or the nurse's manager or mentor can observe. These end-of-program objectives are essentially a description of what the hospital expects a new nurse to be able to do. Sophisticated assessment and intervention do not just appear. Those skills will be developed as the nurse gains experience and becomes socialized into the organization. But the basic knowledge and techniques needed to give safe, effective patient care can be listed in a form that can be used to evaluate orientees—and the success of the orientation program.

In Exhibit 3–2 interim objectives for one specific class are listed. These are more precisely stated objectives, each representing a single activity or learning step. Ultimately these individual objectives lead to the achievement of the overall terminal objectives by orientees. This cumulative impact indicates why you must take as much care in writing the objectives for a single practice session as you do for the program objectives.

Types of Objectives

Learning objectives can be grouped into three major categories: cognitive, psychomotor, and affective. *Cognitive* refers to information and knowledge; *psychomotor* to skills and physical performance; and *affective* to feelings, attitudes, and appreciations. Keeping these three areas in mind may help ensure that some affective objectives are included in the program, since this is the area hardest to measure and thus most easily ignored. But dividing orientation objec-

Exhibit 3–1 Nursing Orientation Objectives

By the end of the three-week orientation, the new nursing employee will be able to:

1. Check in and out on the computer correctly.
2. Locate and use all policy/procedure manuals and guides to determine correct and legal nursing activities.
3. Provide nursing care for a full assignment of patients, including psychosocial assessment and intervention, any teaching required, and all documentation.
4. Correctly and completely document the following:
   a. At least one complete admission, including the admission sheet and note on the clinical record.
   b. At least one discharge, including each of the five required pieces of information about the discharge.
   c. Nurses' notes for several complete shifts, including assessment of the patient at the beginning of the shift, using a systems approach; any nursing activities, treatments, tests, etc., performed; physician visits (by name); patient responses; some teaching done each shift; and the required notes documenting the progress made on the nursing care plan.
   d. All medications administered will be recorded on the M.A.R., including PRN and STAT medications with the required 30-minute follow-up charting.
5. Complete at least three patient care plans and revise at least two others, checking the chart for proper follow-up.

tives into three arbitrary categories seems cumbersome and artificial. A more logical way of approaching the writing of objectives involves setting priorities based on patient care.

Since patients are the reason for a hospital's existence, it makes sense to set priorities for content based on their needs. As you compose program objectives you can be sure of one thing—you will have too much information for the time available. Gillies feels that the most common failing of orientation programs is that too much detailed content is presented to new employees before they feel any need for it.[7]

Objectives help you focus on critical information orientees need in order to give safe, effective care. Take a long, hard look at the content suggested by the needs assessment. What must orientees learn immediately—the first day? What must they know before reaching their department? What should be taught before they actually deal with patients? Anything else does not belong in overall orientation; it should be taught to new employees as they become more familiar with their work place.

Choosing Your Words

Having achieved a rough order of priority, now think about how to describe the competencies that orientees should display to prove they have learned this critical

Exhibit 3–2 Interim Orientation Objectives

Medication Administration and Charting—Objectives

After participating in this session, the participant will be able to:

1. Demonstrate the method of checking the medication book at the beginning of the shift.
2. Explain how the team leader is notified of new orders or changes in orders.
3. Correctly and completely transcribe a medication order into the patient's medication record.
4. Describe or physically perform the following:
   a. Administration of heparin
   b. Intramuscular injection (choice of sites)
   c. Administration of Imferon
5. Explain the nurse's responsibility with regard to controlled drugs.
6. State the preferred way to handle drugs brought from home.
7. Name two medications that can be kept at the bedside with a physician's order.
8. Explain the procedure for correctly documenting drug sensitivities.
9. List the stop order policies for (a) controlled drugs and (b) all other drugs.
10. State what medications require charting on forms other than the medication sheet.

content. Always think in terms of behavior that can be observed and evaluated. For each objective, be sure that:

1. There is an action verb describing what the orientee will do. (The orientee will *send* . . .)
2. There is a description of what materials, equipment, or personnel should be used. (The orientee will send *a carrier through the pneumatic tube system* . . .)
3. There is an unambiguous statement of the level of achievement expected or the criteria that will be used to judge that the objective has been successfully achieved. (The orientee will send a carrier through the pneumatic tube system *so that it reaches an assigned destination*.)

Take a look at the objectives for nursing orientation in Exhibit 3–1. In each case the objective states an action ("check," "locate," "provide," "document," etc.), a description of what will be used ("on the computer," "all policy/procedure manuals and guides," "a full assignment of patients," etc.), and some criterion for evaluation ("correctly," "to determine correct and legal nursing activities," "including psychosocial intervention," etc.).

Each objective must mean exactly the same thing to all other instructors, to all participants, and to the managers and staff who will follow up on the unit. Add enough description to make it clear to everyone concerned just what you expect from orientees. To test if you've achieved this clarity, present the rough draft of the objectives to staff members and ask them to describe what they would expect an orientee to do to demonstrate achievement of each objective.

Individual class objectives should be simpler and shorter. The standards of achievement can sometimes be left to the instructor to define within the context of class activity if that seems appropriate. In Exhibit 3–2 some objectives are stated as instructions (''Explain how the team leader is notified of new orders or changes in orders''), with no criteria listed. Others include criteria (''correctly and completely''). The question to consider when making this judgment is, Will the learner understand what is expected?

Whether writing overall course objectives or individual class objectives, keep your statements as brief and simple as you can make them. Don't feel obligated to include educational jargon or complex conditions of achievement. If you try to make objectives complex or include too much detail, writing them will become an overwhelming chore.

If you have trouble coming up with action verbs, Bloom has developed a complete taxonomy of objectives that divides action verbs into three categories of cognitive, psychomotor, and affective.[8] In most cases, simply thinking about what you expect orientees to do in order to show they have learned what you wanted them to learn is enough to trigger plenty of ideas on how to state the objectives.

COMMUNICATING OBJECTIVES

The list of objectives for orientation should be shared and discussed with all the people involved in orienting new employees. Unless you win agreement from managers and staff, the objectives will be worse than useless—they will mislead new employees by introducing them to one set of standards while they are actually being judged by a totally different set once they reach their respective departments.

Send copies of the objectives to everyone you can think of—and don't forget the administrators who helped with the initial needs assessment. Present the objectives at meetings: managerial meetings (head nurses and department heads), committee meetings (care committees, quality assurance, etc.), and, of course, invite input from members of the Advisory Committee. Before a single orientee has been handed a copy of the objectives, be sure that everyone in the institution remotely likely to work with a new employee has received a copy and understands that these objectives are what will be expected of a new person by the *end* of orientation (not the first day).

CONCLUSION

Instructional objectives are statements describing what the orientee will be able to do by the end of orientation. Stated in terms of behavior that can be observed, they describe orientee performance, not instructor performance or classroom procedures. Writing objectives is easy once the instructor has thought through what new employees need to know in order to function effectively. The statement should be as short and simple as possible. As Mager states, "the purpose of an objective is to communicate something to somebody."[9]

In Chapter 4 the principles of adult education will be related to orientation. The use and misuse of classroom strategies for learning and retention will be presented, including a discussion of the different media that can help or hinder instruction.

NOTES

1. Calvin P. Otto and Rollin O. Glaser, *The Management of Training* (Reading, Mass.: Addison-Wesley Publishing Co., 1970), 342.

2. Martin M. Broadwell, *The Supervisor As An Instructor: A Guide For Classroom Training*, 2d ed. (Reading, Mass.: Addison-Wesley Publishing Co., 1970), 47.

3. Otto and Glaser, *The Management of Training*, 122.

4. *Training and Continuing Education: A Handbook for Health Care Institutions* (Chicago: Hospital Research and Educational Trust, 1970), 36.

5. Robert F. Mager, *Preparing Instructional Objectives*, 2d ed. (Belmont, Calif.: Fearon Publishers, 1975), 5.

6. Jerrold E. Kemp, *Instructional Design* (Belmont, Calif.: Lear Siegler/Fearon Publishers, 1971), 20.

7. Dee Ann Gillies, *Nursing Management: A Systems Approach* (Philadelphia: W.B. Saunders Co., 1982), 207.

8. Benjamin S. Bloom, ed., *Taxonomy of Educational Objectives, Handbook 1* (New York: Longman, 1956).

9. Mager, *Preparing Instructional Objectives*, 68.

Chapter 4

Adult Teaching Techniques

Learning has been defined as "the acquisition of knowledge with subsequent changes in the behavior of the learner."[1] Notice that this definition implies an active process that can only be controlled by the learner, not by the teacher. No one can force another person either to acquire knowledge or to make use of it. An instructor can only provide opportunities for learning and set an atmosphere that encourages the process to take place.

The behavior of the teacher influences the character of the learning climate more than any other single factor.[2] Since hiring is a separate process that usually takes place some time before the first day of employment, the orientation instructor is the first real contact an employee has with the institution. If new workers feel they are treated as responsible adults, respected for their past experience and the knowledge they bring to the new environment, the whole tone of future work relationships is set to positively affect employment.

ADULT EDUCATION PRINCIPLES

Knowles defines *andragogy* as "the art and science of helping adults learn."[3] Andragogy thus incorporates principles different from those of *pedagogy,* the techniques of educating children. As people mature, they develop characteristics unique to adults. If these characteristics are not considered and incorporated in an instructor's approach to adult learners, the teaching efforts will probably fail. It is as inappropriate to treat an adult learner like a child as it would be to require the adult to sit in a chair designed for a first grader. The adult's outlook and approach to learning have grown as much or more than his or her body.

Luckily, a great deal is known about adult learning characteristics, and what is known fits comfortably and appropriately into a hospital orientation program. For instance, adults view themselves as being self-directed and responsible, traits that any employer wants to encourage. Adults have reservoirs of knowledge and experience on which to base new learning, a premise that orientation takes for granted. Most important, adults look for immediate application of information—they want to take what is learned and apply it to the problems they face today, not something that may occur in the future. This has profound implications for ordering content, as well as for reinforcing what is taught in the classroom by practice in the clinical setting.

The problem of what to include in orientation becomes easier to solve if you remember that adults want to learn skills that will help them deal with work situations. "Nice-to-know" information that doesn't directly pertain to what they will be doing tends to bore or distract orientees. Every block of content should be linked to the job; if the relationship is not immediately apparent, point out exactly how the learners will be using the information. If something in the program is not immediately usable, why are you presenting it?

Setting an Adult Learning Climate

The instructor is responsible for maintaining a learning environment that encourages participation and gives orientees a sense of involvement in the learning process. The following guidelines can be used:

1. Make the classroom setup as informal and adult oriented as possible. Everyone should be on the same level (no podiums or stages), and seated so that participants can interact with one another as well as with the instructor. Tables and chairs arranged conference-style or in a U-shape are best. If the only seating you have are chairs with writing arms, arrange them in a semicircle. Avoid the front-facing classroom-style setup—its even rows and formal atmosphere evoke grade school.
2. Establish the fact that you are interested in the orientees as individuals. Have each person give not just name and work area hired into but some details about past work experience and schooling. Then in later discussion you can draw on the background of the group for illustrations and examples.
3. Maintain an atmosphere where participants feel free not only to ask questions but also to disagree. Adults often differ on how things should be done, and they want their opinions heard and considered. By allowing discussion of differences without disapproval, you encourage independent thinking.
4. Adults like some structure and guidance in a learning situation, even if the program is mostly self-study or independent learning. They want to know the "rules" governing the process and, most important, they want to know how they are doing. This does not mean setting up a grading system for orientation—adults tend to resent any evaluation process built on competi-

tion and may withdraw their participation. It does mean building in a series of checkpoints so that learners can assess their progress toward preset objectives. This can be done by ungraded self-tests (''progress checks'' or ''self-assessment'' would be better terms to use) given periodically during the program, perhaps after each block of information. These can be either written or verbal.

5. Adults perceive themselves as able to make decisions and solve problems, so learning experiences that encourage independent thinking and application of information to current problems will be more involving than repetition of facts. Build participation into orientation through case studies, simulations, gaming, and other strategies covered in more detail later in the chapter. One word of caution: many orientees have never been treated as adults in a learning situation and will not be sure how to react when suddenly presented with the opportunity to contribute to their own learning. Be sure to state early in the program that the orientees are responsible for gathering and applying information. This notion of individual learner responsibility may be a new concept for someone used to passively sitting in a classroom listening to an instructor talk. Like any new idea, it takes time to be accepted, so expect some resistance. The best way to overcome it is to make it obvious that applying the information is more useful than writing it down—and more fun, too.

Although learner responsibility has been stressed, this does not mean that the instructor's work is easier. On the contrary, it is more difficult to encourage independent thinking and facilitate application of knowledge than to stand in front of a class and recite facts. Besides demanding constant thought and flexible reactions to the orientees, facilitating adult learning requires a large repertoire of teaching strategies.

STRATEGIES FOR TEACHING ORIENTATION

Experimental research indicates that when learners know what is expected of them they tend to learn regardless of the teaching methods or media used.[4] Why then bother to select and practice different strategies? Because research data also shows that certain teaching strategies are probably more effective for certain learning tasks than others, although these studies are not conclusive.[5] Selection of teaching strategies is far from an exact science. The effectiveness of different methods is always dependent on the teacher's skill and the individuals being taught. Matching the strategy to what needs to be accomplished is the responsibility of the instructor—and what keeps teaching an art as well as a science.

Styles of Learning

One thing to keep in mind when planning what methods to use is that people learn and process information differently. Instructors often act as if everyone learns the way they do—a natural human reaction. However, if you use only teaching strategies that you enjoy, you will not reach some of the participants.

Learning style is defined as "the manner in which an individual perceives and processes information in learning situations."[6] There is a wide range of research available on the topic of learning style identification. Claxton and Ralston organized learning style findings into two basic categories: (1) research that focuses on observing how people perceive and respond to stimuli in their environments (cognitive style) and (2) research that grows out of psychological tests and observations of how students behave and interact in the classroom (student response style).[7]

Samples of cognitive styles include *field independent-dependent,* which involves the ability to perceive items without being influenced by the background, or *preceptive/receptive-systematic/intuitive,* which examines information gathering and evaluation.[8] Student response styles focus on student reactions to learning, classroom procedures, teachers, and peers. The Grasha-Reichmann model identifies the dimensions as (1) *independent-dependent,* (2) *collaborative-competitive,* and (3) *participant-avoidant.*[9]

Integrated models incorporate learning theory, individual development, and personality types. An example of these eclectic models is the Kolb Learning Style Inventory, which describes four different approaches to learning:

1. *Converger*—likes a single correct solution to a problem and enjoys dealing with things rather than people.
2. *Diverger*—likes situations that call for generation of ideas and is interested in people.
3. *Assimilator*—likes to create theoretical models and is less interested in people and more concerned with abstract concepts.
4. *Accommodator*—likes doing things such as carrying out plans and experiments and relies heavily on other people for information rather than on own analytic ability.[10]

Obviously, one teaching method will not reach all types of learners. A lecture would probably be well accepted by a converger, but a diverger would be bored by it. Role playing would be effective for accommodators and divergers, but neither assimilators nor convergers would enjoy or learn from it.

Rezler and Rezmovic constructed the Learning Preference Inventory (LPI) to identify preferred modes of learning by health professionals. It includes six scales: Abstract, Concrete, Individual, Interpersonal, Student-structured, and Teacher-structured.[11] Assessment of learning preferences helps match participants with learning conditions that they find rewarding. Even if you find it impractical to test every group of orientees, it is obvious that a range of teaching methods should be used during orientation to reach all learners—and also to expose the participants to new ways of learning. Remember, if you rely on one or two approaches that are comfortable and have worked well in the past, you may not be reaching part of your audience.

Selecting Teaching Strategies

The key to selecting any teaching method is to target the objectives. In order to present information effectively, instructors must choose strategies based on the objectives they wish to achieve. There are three basic patterns for teaching and learning: presentation, independent study, and teacher-student interaction. Each can be used effectively to achieve instructional objectives. Presentations (lecture, film, demonstration) offer information that relates to cognitive and psychomotor objectives. Independent study (reading, programmed learning, problem solving) achieves cognitive and psychomotor objectives and is occasionally helpful in promoting affective ones. Interaction (questioning, group work, discussion) is especially useful for affective objectives, although it can apply to all three types.[12]

If the objective concerns the acquisition of knowledge, design learning experiences that will help the orientees build associations between new information and their present knowledge. Providing learners with time to review and translate the information into their own words ensures that it will be remembered later on.

If the objective relates to skill acquisition, the strategies chosen should pattern the techniques to be learned as closely as possible. The more concrete classroom learning and practice is, the more easily the skill will translate to the working environment.

Affective objectives require active involvement of the learners in questioning and supporting different views. Although orientation may not seem to call for a large number of affective objectives, the ones that may be involved are usually very important. For example, if you are introducing the concept of primary nursing to newly hired nurses, it would be crucial for each orientee to accept the values inherent in this type of nursing practice. If a nurse did not agree, for instance, with the idea of 24-hour responsibility for patients, all the knowledge and skills in the world would not make this particular learner a successful primary nurse.

Table 4–1 can be used as a guide for choosing different techniques based on the objectives you wish to achieve. Notice that some techniques can be used for different aims. Each of these strategies will be discussed in detail later in the chapter.

Table 4–1 Teaching Techniques for Achieving Objectives

	Objectives	
Cognitive	*Psychomotor*	*Affective*
Lecture	Demonstration	Discussion
Question/Answer	Tours	Question/Answer
Discussion	Simulations	Tours
Tours	Action projects	Guest speakers
Guest speakers	Experiments	Case studies
Self-studies	Observations	Simulations
Action projects	Checklists	Role playing
Books	Hands-on practice	Action projects
Gaming	Clinical practice	Gaming

Linton and Truelove list other factors besides achievement of objectives that should be considered when choosing a teaching technique:

1. Trainees' previous education, experience, interest, and motivation.
2. Degree of content difficulty and complexity.
3. Class size.
4. Availability and cost of facilities and equipment.
5. Training time—most efficient and effective method for allocated time.[13]

Assessing individual and group preparation and readiness to learn requires experience. Obviously, a group of laypeople to be trained as unit secretaries needs to be approached differently than a group of registered nurses being oriented to the facility. But even within that seemingly homogeneous group of nurses there may be radically different levels of education and experience. Examining hiring records illuminates some of these differences, but only individual interviews or in-class interactions will reveal each participant's interest in learning the information you have to present. Instructors have enormous impact on learner motivation through the interest they show in each person in the class. If you make it clear you want each member to learn and are willing to help in any way you can, orientees will respond. Flexibility in the use of teaching techniques based on learning style and preparation of group members is one way to demonstrate your concern.

The degree of content complexity also dictates your approach. Instructing someone on how to use the hospital phone system calls for a simple explanation, demonstration, and return demonstration. But a subject such as assessing patients' reactions to drugs requires careful consideration of previous learner knowledge, presentation of the content in several different ways, and a built-in evaluation of how the information has been received and processed. This evaluation must be done in class by the instructor in order to ensure that all members of the group know how to react appropriately to an adverse drug reaction. Methods for evaluating learning complex content include quizzes immediately following content presentation, questions asked at several points during the experience, case studies simulating patient situations, or a formal written examination.

The size of group has a profound impact on the teaching techniques chosen. If you have decided to let each person explain and demonstrate how different pieces of equipment are used, the group will probably learn about the equipment discussed, particularly if each person can handle each piece after it has been explained. For a group of seven orientees this would be an excellent teaching strategy. Try the same approach with a group of 30 people—even if you adapt it so that group members demonstrate the equipment in front of the class and then everyone is allowed to pick up the equipment and examine it, the immediacy and one-to-one interchange is gone. Within that group of 30, at least one person (you will be lucky if there is only one) will not have learned the correct way to use that equipment. Some other strategy should be chosen—perhaps equipment review for a group that large could be done on the units.

Equipment availability and cost is a growing problem. The instructor who has a wide range of manikins, materials, and audio-visual equipment at hand has many more options available than the instructor who can barely obtain a classroom and chairs. Sometimes lack of equipment can be remedied. Put the most badly needed piece in the budget request, along with an eloquent justification. If you don't request what you need, the institution won't know you need it. In the meantime, use ingenuity to work around the lack of equipment—many of the strategies to be discussed require no expensive hardware.

The final criterion for choosing teaching techniques—effective use of training time—may be the most important of all except targeting the objectives. As budget restrictions have more and more impact on hospital operations, people involved in hospital education must begin to assess their practice not only by how well it worked but also by how much it cost. How efficient is each method? Cantor states: "The fact that educational material is accurate, interesting, and even generally relevant does not mean it is necessarily appropriate for a given purpose or is the most efficient means of presenting content."[14] As each strategy is discussed below, some mention will be made of its cost effectiveness.

Lecture

Lecturing is perhaps the most misused and misunderstood of all teaching methods; it also is the approach people have experienced most often. Throughout formal schooling lecture is widely used, which accounts for a built-in disadvantage when the learner enters the work force. To many people the beginning of a lecture signals a return to school, and adults may resent this feeling. Frequently the lecture method is criticized because it places students in a passive role, but this will happen only if you let it. Lecturing can be a superb teaching strategy—if planned and executed properly.

First of all, a lecture should never be used to deliver facts. If the orientees need to learn a block of information, let them read a handout or procedure book. Recent studies have shown that the lecture can be used effectively to help students develop the ability to apply concepts and to generalize, so use lecturing as a way of relating information to the overall picture, of clarifying difficult relationships.[15] As an example of how lecture can accomplish this, during a class on cardiopulmonary resuscitation (CPR), a nurse asked what actually happened physiologically during a myocardial infarction. The answer was a minilecture on the mechanics and pathophysiology involved. When it was completed, the entire class of ten RNs stated that this was the first time they had really understood what happened within the cardiopulmonary system as a heart attack was taking place. These were all experienced medical-surgical nurses. How many times had they studied this subject? Yet something in that impromptu lecture tied it all together for them in a way that nothing else ever had. That light of comprehension—the "ah-hah!"—kindling in someone's expression makes it well worthwhile preparing lectures carefully.

Preparing the Lecture

Unless you are completely familiar with the topic, research is the first step in preparing the lecture. How you go about it depends on the content. If the lecture is designed to clarify how something is done at your hospital, research would involve not only knowing the procedure but also actually having done it. Talk to people who perform it every day. What problems can arise? How are they handled? Watch the procedure being done. What individual differences do you see? Do these differences have any impact on the effectiveness of the procedure?

Researching a theoretical topic such as legal implications of nursing is more involved. Obviously, resources in the literature will be studied and notes taken on the information garnered from these books and articles. It is when these notes are being put together in lecture form that problems often develop. Novice instructors usually string their notes together into a written speech that consists of one quote after another. There are two reasons not to do this: first, a lecturer who presents material taken wholly from resources *does not know the information*. No one expects you to know every topic off the top of your head—research is always required. But once you have studied the books and articles, make the data collected your own. Play with it in your mind. What does it mean? How does each piece of information relate to the others? How do you perceive the whole concept in relationship to its parts? What problems do you have with it? Your students will probably have the same ones.

The best way to test your comprehension is to state the concept in your own words, without reference to any notes. If you can bring your own ideas and unique interpretation to the facts, you will be able to help participants relate the information to their own personal knowledge and experience. Being able to understand concepts also prepares you to handle questions, no matter how "off the wall" some of them may be.

The second reason for not writing the lecture word for word is also very practical: you will find yourself chained to your manuscript. Participants don't like to be read to—they know how to read. Using a written script makes it hard to react spontaneously to student questions, comments, and body language. If you deliver the lecture using only brief notes you can adapt the actual words you use to the reactions of the group. To gain confidence, go ahead and write the lecture out if it will help fix the thoughts firmly in mind. Just never take it into the classroom.

Most seasoned instructors prepare their notes as a tool to keep them on target during lectures. The key word in using notes is *brevity:* the fewer notes, the better your delivery. Their function is to give you an organized plan to follow. Outline the presentation and reduce the outline to key words. Exhibit 4–1 illustrates a sample note card for a lecture on assessment of the central nervous system. Some instructors find it helpful to color code their notes—activities underlined in red, audio-visual aids in blue, handouts in green, for instance. Others use symbols such as arrows, boxes, or asterisks to key in student and teacher activities. Use whatever proves helpful, but be sure to standardize your system and use the same thing every time.

Exhibit 4–1 Note Card for Lecture on Assessment of the Central Nervous System

C. MOTOR SYSTEM ASSESSMENT

1. Test for *drift* (demonstrate)
2. Note involuntary movement (see handout for 6 abnormalities)
3. Check for *clonus* (SLIDE)
4. Coordination tests—*cerebellar* dysfunction
    a. Finger-to-nose (eyes open/closed)
    b. Heel-to-shin
    c. Alternating movements
5. Balance
    a. Check for *Romberg's sign* (demonstrate)
    b. Stay close to prevent fall
6. Gait
    a. Review abnormal gaits (SLIDES)
    b. Discuss nursing implications

Rehearsing the Lecture

Beware of memorization. Not only will it make your presentation flat and dull but all it takes is one moment of forgetfulness to ruin your entire performance. One expert on presentation skills states that "Thinking is the first principle of good rehearsal."[16] Therefore, your first action in the rehearsal process is to think through the lecture, point by point. This will doublecheck the organization and internal consistency and enable you to decide what points to emphasize and how you will do it. Once this initial analysis is done, rehearse by

1. Working from the notes you have made from your outline to be sure those key words trigger your memory.
2. Memorizing your opening and closing statements.
3. Testing key transitions and different wordings by saying them aloud.
4. Practicing with any teaching aids (flipchart, overhead transparencies, audio-visual equipment, etc.) to be sure you can handle them smoothly.
5. Using the room where the actual lecture will be delivered. This helps in planning setup and movement.

Some lecturers practice by recording their presentation on audiotape. If you try this, listen for vocal quality and clear enunciation as well as content. But don't use the tape player repeatedly—it's a sure lure to memorizing the lecture.

Delivering the Lecture

Introduce each lecture by outlining the key points that will be covered. In addition to emphasizing what should be remembered this overview helps students grasp the total topic. Encouraging participants to focus on important points should be a major goal. After two days most people forget at least 75 percent of what they have heard.[17] Repeat the information in several different ways. Just making the same statement over and over again will not help, so use a visual aid, ask a question, tell an illustrative anecdote—make the repetitions count.

Information should progress logically and smoothly with frequent pauses for feedback. Watch for nonverbal clues such as glancing around, yawning, looking at watches or the room clock. If group members demonstrate boredom or discomfort, vary the routine. Give an unscheduled break, start an activity that gets them up and moving, or have them stand, stretch, and take some deep breaths. You might also ask the group if they're already familiar with this information or are perhaps merely tired.

Contributing to the problem of student restlessness and boredom are two sins instructors commit with great frequency: content overload and lengthy class sessions. It's especially tempting to pack too much content into orientation classes. There's so much that needs to be covered and so little time to cover it. But presenting large amounts of information without giving participants time to think about the data leads to anxiety, exhaustion, and ultimate lack of retention. Limit content to essentials, and allow enough time for frequent pauses, so that participants can manipulate the information and fit it into their own mental framework. Provide chances for the orientees to test their grasp of the material by short tests on what has been covered (see Exhibit 4–2 for sample review questions). After the first few quizzes you may find the orientees listening more carefully to the information presented. Needless to say, these tests are never graded, since they are used for review and retention.

Class length is an important consideration. Expecting people to sit and listen to a lecture for eight hours, even with breaks and lunch, is cruel and inhumane. If you must have full-day classes, individual and group activities should be built into the schedule. The longest that any group should be expected to sit is 90 minutes. Remember that people are generally fresher in the morning, especially after the first break. After lunch is the worst time for lecture—everyone can remember the heavy-lidded feeling as digestion draws blood from the brain. Always get participants on their feet and moving after lunch, and go easy on the lecturing in the afternoon, as everyone gets more and more tired.

Cost Effectiveness

Lecturing is very cost effective, since the same presentation can be made to large groups as easily as small ones. It can also be repeated many times at no cost increase. Most people are familiar with lecture and feel comfortable with it as a teaching method, and those learners who are analytical and theory oriented find it one of the most efficient ways of learning.

Exhibit 4–2 Sample Review Questions

Medication Administration

1. List the three types of drugs that can be left at the patient's bedside (with a physician's order):
   a.
   b.
   c.
2. Describe how the Medication Administration Record is checked against the Kardex at the beginning of each shift:

The burden of responsibility for lecture effectiveness falls on the instructor. Prepare carefully, maintain eye contact, watch for feedback, and project your own interest in the subject. Summaries of research on teaching effectiveness consistently cite qualities such as warmth, enthusiasm, and motivation.[18]

Questioning

Asking Questions of the Group

Many adults are reluctant to speak up in class. This can be due to past experiences where a teacher reacted negatively to an answer or fellow learners sighed or snickered at some response—both devastating experiences. Participants may fear that their answer will be wrong or sound silly. Thus, even when most people in the group know the answer, you may have trouble eliciting a response to questions. The following strategies may help get those answers:

1. Make questions nonthreatening. Stress the fact that you want to check whether your explanations are clear, or to get input from the group—not that you want to see if they've been paying attention.
2. Be sure everyone can hear the question, and phrase it simply. Don't ask three different things within the same question; no one will be sure which you want answered.
3. Show interest in the answer. Lean forward with your eyes fixed on the speaker and concentrate on what's being said. One of the motives for speaking up in class is to gain attention, so be attentive.
4. Find something valuable in every response. Even if it's not the answer you were hoping for, the participant has invested some ego in it, so support it with some statement like "That's an interesting point."
5. The most important technique to use when asking questions is: WAIT FOR THE ANSWER. Novices frequently make the mistake of becoming uncomfortable with silence after a question has been asked. Jumping in with your own answer or with a restatement of the question cuts off any response and conditions the group not to answer your questions. Let the silence grow. Wait them out, no matter how long it takes, all the while looking around expectantly. Sooner or later one of the participants will speak, if only to ask you to clarify the question. Be patient.

Answering Group Questions

Who hasn't heard a teacher say "Be sure to stop me if you have any questions" and then proceed to rattle through the presentation at breakneck speed? If you want people to ask questions (and you should, in order to check understanding), you must encourage them to do so. It's not enough just to ask for questions at the end of the session. Besides stating that you want them to interrupt if they have a question, pause for questions at 10- to 15-minute intervals. When doing this:

1. Repeat every question before you answer it, both to clarify your own comprehension and to be sure everyone heard it.
2. If you don't know the answer, don't fake it. Say something like "I don't know the answer to that one. How can we find it?" Let the group help you problem solve, but be sure you get the answer and report back.
3. Watch for puzzled expressions and check them out by saying "You look as if you'd like more information on that point," or "Would you like an example?"
4. Watch for questions. That sounds obvious, but many teachers say "Any questions?" while arranging their next transparency or looking at their notes. It takes an assertive student to say aloud "Yes, I have a question."
5. Allow time for questions. If you ask for questions, pause a beat, and then launch into the next section of the lecture, it's not surprising that none are forthcoming.
6. Don't show impatience. Even if what is being asked was covered two minutes ago, give the questioner the benefit of the doubt and assume he or she didn't understand, rather than didn't listen. Any indication that the instructor considers a question stupid or useless freezes other participants into immobility. No one wants to be put down in front of his or her peers—or see the same thing happen to another student.

Questioning is the most effective method known for eliciting feedback and clarifying misunderstandings. Let it work for you.

Discussion

A discussion is an exchange of feelings and opinions. When beginning a period of discussion, the first thing an instructor must do is establish why this discussion is necessary. Why is precious class time being spent on it? Some instructors break people up into small groups for discussion whenever they run out of things to say. This shouldn't happen in orientation, but beware of using discussion when it isn't needed. Participants tend to resent wasting time this way.

When leading a discussion, the most important thing to do is *listen*. Concentrate on responses and use them to keep the discussion flowing and to stimulate responses from other group members. For instance, use a statement by a vocal person to encourage someone who hasn't contributed by saying "What do you think about that response?" or "How does that fit in with your experience?" (Don't use questions that can be answered yes or no.) Learning takes place in a discussion when participants are made to think.

If the purpose of the discussion is to gather ideas, keep a record of responses on a chalkboard or flipchart. End the session with a summary of what has been discussed, and provide a definite conclusion. Participants appreciate a sense of closure.

Small Group Format

Use small groups when the total group is too large for everyone to participate freely. Some experts recommend a maximum number of 15.[19] In many cases that large a group seems to block input from the less assertive members. Six seems to be optimum small group membership, with eight still working well. Over that number, you will often find that some members will not participate. Arrange the groups in circles and give them clear instructions on what they are to accomplish and how long they have to accomplish it. Each group should select a spokesperson to report its findings to the total group.

Cost Effectiveness

Discussion works well to help orientees explore feelings about issues and brainstorm solutions to problems. It is not an efficient method for learning content. When setting discussion time aside in orientation, be sure it will accomplish objectives; otherwise the time would be better spent in some other activity.

Demonstrations

Demonstrating a procedure is unparalleled for teaching concrete tasks and skills. Watching the actual equipment used properly is hard to beat as a teaching method. The close correlation between the learning situation and on-the-job performance heightens learner interest and motivation.

Demonstration requires careful preparation. Before class begins, be sure each piece of equipment works, and run through the procedure several times, no matter how well you know it. If a demonstration doesn't go well, it will do more harm than good. Arrange the group so that all members have a clear view of whatever you are demonstrating. If the technique requires them to see fine adjustments of dials or meters, a taped demonstration with appropriate close-ups will be more effective than a live one.

As you demonstrate the procedure, emphasize the sequence of steps and key performance points. Explain the reasoning behind such sequencing, and involve the group by asking how they see this procedure being used in their work area. A demonstration is always most effective if observers are allowed to practice the skill immediately after having seen it performed. If time, space, or lack of equipment prevent return demonstrations, at least be sure group members can manipulate the equipment during a break or after class. Try to ensure clinical follow-up by arranging for them to perform the demonstrated procedure as soon as possible in their departments.

Cost Effectiveness

Although extremely effective in teaching skills, demonstrations require time and equipment that can make this a costly teaching method. If the group is large, demonstrations are best done on an individual basis in work areas, since inability to see the procedure renders it useless.

Guest Speakers

Having people from different departments speak to orientees is an old orientation tradition. New employees are introduced to key people in the hospital, thus aiding socialization to the new environment. Familiarity with the speakers' departments and how the orientees' areas interact with them fosters greater interdepartmental communication and understanding.

To avoid inundating orientees with guest speakers, the orientation instructor must apply some ruthless guidelines:

1. What purpose will be served by having this information delivered by this particular person? If the director of nursing explains the organization of the nursing department to new nurses, they not only receive the information but also begin a valuable acquaintance with an important leader. The director achieves familiarity with new employees and their goals and interests. By any criterion, this guest speaker is an effective choice.
2. Can the speaker deliver information effectively? An uncomfortable speaker reading a prepared speech in a monotone will accomplish nothing. Unless the person can come across as an experienced, knowledgeable professional with useful information, choose someone else or some other method of delivery.
3. Is there time for the objective to be accomplished by a guest speaker? In orientation one always comes back to time—there is never enough. Although the Radiology Department may want to speak to new employees about preparing patients for radiologic procedures, a simple handout of instructions may be more efficient, and the information possibly better retained, than a speech prepared by the department head. Saying no takes tact, but it may be necessary.

Cost Effectiveness

Utilizing guest speakers is rarely cost effective because of the high salaries of the people involved and most speakers' tendency to ramble over the allotted time.

Unless there is a secondary reason for using a guest speaker (as in the value of interacting with an administrator, discussed above), other methods of delivering information should be chosen.

Case Studies/Simulations

Case studies and simulations are representations of a real situation or process. Participants are required to apply previously learned knowledge to respond to the problem and receive feedback about their decisions.[20] Case studies and simulations can be used to sharpen decision-making skills, develop proficiency in interpersonal relationships, and solve real-life problems without real-life consequences.

Don't use simulations or case studies just to fill time or provide entertainment. They should accomplish specific objectives. Exhibit 4–3 is an example of a simple case study that asks nursing participants to assess patient reactions to drug regimens and decide what actions should be taken. Simulations and case studies

Exhibit 4–3 Sample Case Studies

Bill J. is a 76-year-old admitted for treatment of mild CHF and senility. He has been on your unit for two days now. He is 5′10″, 140 lbs., and this AM his V.S. were: T. 97.2, P. 72, R 24, B/P 130/90. He is on a regular diet, but this morning says that he doesn't feel like eating. The NA stated that Mr. J. didn't want to help with AM care either, saying he felt "too tired." When you walk into the room, he calls you "Janet" and says he "has to go feed the dogs."

His drug regime includes:

Digoxin 0.25 mg. p.o. daily
Slow-K 1 BID
M.O.M. 30 cc. HS PRN
Hydrodiuril 50 mg. BID
Seconal 100 mg. HS

Barbara C. is a 32-year-old admitted for a cholecystectomy. Three days post-op she developed a temperature of 102. She has been treated for a wound infection for the past four days. When you go in to change her dressing you notice that the drainage seems normal and the wound edges clean. She states that she feels "much better" except for the diarrhea that started last night and is still bothering her. "I have to go every five minutes," she says. "Could you ask the doctor to order some Lomotil? That always works for me."

Her drug regimen includes:

Clindamycin HC1 300 mg. IM q. 6 hrs.
Meperidine 50 mg. IM q. 3–4 hrs. PRN for severe pain
Percodan 1–2 tabs. p.o. q. 3–4 hrs. for mild to moderate pain
ASA gr. X P.O. q. 4 hrs. PRN for temp. over 100
Decholin 250 mg. p.o. TID p.c.
Nembutal 100 mg. P.O. HS PRN

can be short or very long and detailed. Whether short or long, the case should provide a clear picture of certain people and events.

Although professionally written cases are available, individualized studies are often more effective because the instructor can tailor them to the institution and its policies. Keep your focus on what you want the simulated experience to accomplish as you follow these steps:

1. Outline the case, and decide whether you want it to contain irrelevant details by asking "Should the participants be able to distinguish between necessary and unnecessary data?"
2. Decide what situations should be included.
3. Write the entire case in detail. Be sure to include enough information to enable participants to analyze the situation.
4. Ask questions designed to get feedback about the process. What decisions were made? Was all information considered? What do the participants feel they did wrong? What did they learn from the process?

Cost Effectiveness

Although highly effective for developing decision-making skills and helpful for problem solving and analysis, case studies and simulations can be time consuming and expensive. Cost is kept down by writing your own cases, but an instructor who takes a long time to write each simulation will raise costs through labor expenses. Even if efficiently written and reproduced, any simulation takes a good deal of class time to work through.

Role Playing

Role playing is a technique in which some problem involving human interaction is presented and then spontaneously acted out.[21] The situation should be work related and should include just enough detail to involve the participants in what will happen. No role-playing situation will ever happen exactly the same way twice; this creative development heightens excitement for the instructor as well as for the participants.

Writing a role play is similar to writing case studies, but the problems should involve communication breakdowns or other relational difficulties. The instructor works hard during role playing. If the stage is improperly set, participants may treat the whole thing as a joke. To properly prepare the group:

1. Don't begin a class with role play; the orientees need to become acquainted and feel comfortable with each other.

2. Choose an important problem and be sure your introduction is serious and focused on problem resolution.
3. Give players time to prepare for the role.
4. Give the observers something to do: report, evaluate, or referee.
5. Conduct a post-play discussion to highlight what was learned from the role play.

Cost Effectiveness

Role plays are not easy to do well. They require careful supervision and debriefing by the instructor. Some adult learners are uncomfortable with role playing and will react negatively to it, blocking potential learning. And it is time consuming, so it may be an expensive method for achieving objectives. However, content covered during a role play will often be remembered by participants far longer than that learned using more conventional teaching methods.

Gaming

A game designed to facilitate learning should be based on real-life situations and should contain rules, goals, sets of activities to perform, constraints on what can be done, and payoffs as consequences for player behavior.[22] Many learners like a gaming format, and competition heightens motivation to learn the information.

Before trying to compose a game, participate in several of the commercial ones to get a feel for the gaming process. Examples of already prepared games include "The Quality Assurance Game" (Medical Education Associates, 16792 Madrone Circle, Fountain Valley, California 92708), a board game designed to introduce health care professionals to the process of setting up a hospitalwide quality assurance system; and "Hospitex" (Management Games, Ltd., 11 Woburn St., Ampthill, Bedford, England, MK45 2HP), a game designed to teach nurses the skills and techniques necessary to take charge of a nursing unit.

To design your own game:

1. Decide on the game's purpose. What do you want the participants to come away with when they finish the game?
2. Write specific objectives for the game. These should be shared with the participants.
3. Based on your overall purpose and objectives, decide on the structure of the game: board format, cards, interactional.
4. Plan the sequence of play, the rules and constraints, and the criteria for "winning." How many people can play at the same time? How much equipment or materials are required? How long will it take to play? Limit the number of players, keep the rules and playing sequence as simple as

possible, and limit the materials you have to make. Although there is no set rule for length of play, participants need to spend long enough at it to become involved, but not so long as to become bored. Keep the play fast moving and you won't have to worry about length.

5. The most carefully planned section of the game should involve debriefing. The discussion of what happened during play is crucial to stimulating participants to think about what was learned.
6. Test your game by asking some colleagues to play it. This is the only way to discover the bugs inevitably present in any game. Revise the structure based on feedback from other instructors and your own feelings about how the process went.

Exhibit 4–4 is a simple game used in orientation to teach the location of crash cart equipment.

Exhibit 4–4 Game Used in Orientation

"Beat the Clock"

Locate the following:
Oxygen flowmeter
500 cc NaCl
18 gauge IV cannula
IV tubing
Suction catheter
Curved laryngoscope blade
Ambu bag
Sodium bicarbonate
Metriset
#7 endotracheal tube
Subclavian set
10 cc syringe
Tape
Hemostat
Cutdown tray
Lubricant
Extra batteries
ABG tray
3-way stopcock
Ampule of epinephrine
Tourniquet
Tracheotomy tray
Extension tube

Score:
5 minutes—"Oh, oh"
4 minutes—"Review cart"
3 minutes—"Pretty good"
2 minutes—"Wow!"
1 minute —"Supernurse!"

Cost Effectiveness

Playing a game can help instructors assess how well orientees transfer knowledge to on-the-job skills. Game experts agree that the closer a game's structure simulates reality the more likely and extensive the transfer of learning.[23] If the cost of materials and trainee/instructor time is kept down, gaming can be cost as well as learning effective.

Self-Studies

Perhaps the fastest-growing approach to orienting new employees is the use of self-study. Advantages include (1) placing accountability for learning with the learners, (2) acknowledging that adults are self-directing, and (3) letting the learners work at their own pace.

In orientation programs self-study has generally been implemented through use of learning contracts in which employees agree to master specific content within an agreed-on time. Criteria for mastery are negotiated by each individual employee and the instructor or manager; these criteria can be modified if problems arise. There are many different types of learning contracts and each hospital should probably design its own, being sure to include the following:

1. Instructional objectives that are learner specific.
2. Resources and learning strategies available.
3. Time limits.
4. How achievement will be evaluated: what evidence indicates that the knowledge or skill has been attained? Periodic progress reports keep track of learner activities and enable you to offer assistance before serious problems arise.

Besides using the obvious resources such as policy and procedure books and handouts, methods of self-study include action projects carried out on the unit (such as developing a care plan for a certain type of patient), independent research using the hospital library, and perhaps the most familiar of all—programmed instruction. (See Exhibit 4–5 for an excerpt from a programmed study.)

Programmed Instruction

Programmed instruction can be produced completely in written form, or presented in combination with audio-visual aids or equipment. Learners progressing through a programmed study receive information in a series of small steps called frames, each of which requires a short response about the information in the last frame. Only after giving a correct response can learners proceed to the next frame. The two types of programmed instruction are called *linear* and *branching*. Linear

Exhibit 4–5 Excerpt from Programmed Study

ADVERSE REACTIONS TO DRUGS AND RELATED SUBSTANCES

OVER 10% OF PATIENTS WHO RECEIVE INDICATED DRUGS EXPERIENCE UNFORESEEN ADVERSE EFFECTS FROM THEIR MEDICATION.

Fever is a feature of many drug reactions and occasionally is the sole manifestation of an adverse response. Since both granulocytes and monocytes release substances that indirectly elevate body temperature, it is not surprising that fever accompanies a variety of processes. Drug-related fever has been noted particularly with penicillin, sulfanomides, iodide, streptomycin, Dilantin, and others.

(PLEASE TURN TO THE NEXT PAGE.)

QUESTIONS

1. What percentage of patients will suffer from adverse drug reactions?

   10%

2. List two drugs that might cause the patient to run a fever.

   PENICILLIN, SULFANOMIDES, IODIDE, STREPTOMYCIN, DILANTIN

Drug-associated circulating complexes are known to facilitate RBC, leukocyte, and platelet destruction in certain instances. These occurrences have been associated with quinidine, the anti-TB drugs, and sulfanomides. Initially, complexes of host IgG or IgM and drug (or drug-related protein conjugates) become attached to one or more blood cell types. Complement components are localized to the cell surface as a result, and their interaction results in discrete membrane lesions or rapid removal from the circulation, the formed elements being injured as "innocent bystanders."

(PLEASE TURN TO THE NEXT PAGE.)

instruction proceeds from frame to frame, covering simple material with the correct answer shown in an adjacent frame. The branching method offers multiple-choice answers. When an incorrect response is made, the learner is instructed to turn to a section that explains the information in a different way. This branch must be completed correctly before the learner moves on to new material.

Writing programmed instruction is difficult and time consuming. Several professional journals present occasional programmed learning modules that readers complete for continuing education credit. Look at some of these as examples of what can be accomplished with this method. If an individualized program is needed, be sure to:

1. Write clear objectives for the program to accomplish.
2. Break down the information into easily comprehended segments.
3. Compose questions and answers that give the learner immediate feedback.

4. Test the program on instructors and trainees both, to validate the progression of information and evaluation.
5. Write a pretest and post-test to measure the degree to which the desired learning is taking place (see Exhibit 4–6).

Computer Assisted Instruction (CAI)

The newest method of conducting self-study is through use of computer terminals. Using the principles of programmed instruction, participants learn information piece by piece and answer questions asked periodically by the program. The computer responds to the answers with praise or correction and invites the learner

---

Exhibit 4–6 Post-Test for Programmed Study

FINAL QUESTIONS

1. What percentage of patients suffer from adverse drug reactions?

   10%

2. Penicillin, iodide, and/or Dilantin might cause elevated __________.

   TEMPERATURE

3. List what element of the blood is damaged or diminished in the following:
   a. Agranulocytosis (leukopenia)—LEUKOCYTES (WBC)
   b. Hemolysis—RED BLOOD CELLS
   c. Thrombocytopenia—PLATELETS

4. Adverse respiratory effects may be caused by what drug?

   NITROFURANTOIN

(PLEASE GO TO THE NEXT PAGE.)

5. What penicillin can be especially dangerous to the kidneys?

   METHICILLIN

6. Erythromycin can cause cholestasis with what accompanying symptom?

   JAUNDICE

7. By far the largest proportion of adverse drug reactions involve the ?

   SKIN

8. What can occur if the offending medication is not withdrawn?

   EXFOLIATIVE DERMATITIS WITH SKIN SHEDDING

9. What can the appearance of *firm* hemorrhagic spots mean?

   INFLAMMATORY LESIONS OF THE SMALL BLOOD VESSELS, OR INVOLVEMENT OF DIVERSE ORGANS.

(THE END)

to proceed. These responses make CAI a more personalized method of learning than the written self-studies.

There are a few computer programs designed specifically for hospital employees, but software is generally limited. Companies supplying the equipment have courses available to teach instructors to write their own programs. Computer assisted instruction should have many applications to orientation, since much of the information is fact based and repetitive. In the future new employees may control orientation through pacing and interaction with selected computer programs. Terminals can be placed in different areas of the hospital so that learners have easy access to information at any time of the day or night. People could be oriented directly onto their shift of choice without suffering through daytime classes and rearranging their schedules.

Cost Effectiveness

The self-study approach is based on the principles of adult education: self-direction, individualization, structured learning opportunities, frequent feedback. Although no substitute for individual attention by managers and instructors, self-study offers an attractive alternative to traditional classes. Costs can be kept down by developing programs quickly; usually the more you compose, the easier it gets. Eliminating repetition of the same content saves instructor salaries. If orientees absorb and retain information more efficiently through self-study, there may even be savings in participant salaries.

Self-study through computers makes orientation flexible and learner controlled. Incoming young employees will be familiar with computer use and comfortable with this method of learning. Remember that the initial outlay for computer equipment may be in the range of $20,000 to $40,000. If several hospitals in the same area are willing to share the cost, most systems can function through phone-line communications. Such resource sharing makes hard economic sense.

Audio-Visual Media

Over 60 percent of the information received by a learner is visual.[24] It only makes sense that audio-visual support for presentations increases attention and retention. However, avoid indiscriminate use of these aids. Too many flipcharts, slides, handouts, and other visual keys lead to sensory overload and confusion. A common trap for inexperienced instructors is to create audio-visuals rather than to support objectives. To avoid this, Mambert suggests asking three questions:

1. Does this idea need support or reinforcement?
2. Of the methods available, which is the best?
3. How can I make every element of this support contribute?[25]

Keep in mind that audio-visual aids should be used to clarify ideas that cannot be adequately explained in words alone. They work best when the message comes across in one single visual punch. With any of the aids discussed, remember these general guidelines:

1. Never let an aid stand alone. Introduce it by pointing out what participants should get from the aid—the purpose or objective.
2. Limit aids to the main points of the presentation so that these are highlighted by visual as well as verbal impact. If you use aids to enhance every part of the information, the students will wind up remembering nothing.
3. Reinforce the points made in several different ways.
4. Debrief participants after using an aid to be sure the point was understood (ask questions, generate discussion, or conduct a short quiz).

Actual Objects

Most audio-visual experts agree that the actual object is the best aid of all.[26] Orientation groups work with actual chart forms, real equipment, and other materials from the work environment. Using the real thing enhances transfer of learning to the world of work. If the actual object is too hard to transport or impractical to use (a Clinitron bed, the hospital computer system, real patients), create working models or illustrations. Heavy equipment can enter the classroom via detailed pictures and diagrams. Biomedical engineering can develop a mockup of computer terminals or other hospital systems that orientees can manipulate. Patients can be replaced with role-playing instructors or participants for in-class interviews; and for situations requiring student action, various manikins are available—Resusci-Annie for CPR is the most famous.

The major disadvantage of using actual objects is the expense of the materials. Most things can be recycled for repeated use after cleaning and repair, and the high transfer of learning seems worth it in most cases. Another factor to keep in mind is safety. Screen participants carefully before allowing them to use equipment that could exacerbate physical problems. For example, Exhibit 4–7 is a list of instructions given to participants attending a CPR class.

Handouts

The first thing to ask when deciding whether or not to prepare a handout is "Is this really necessary?" Handouts are overused by instructors and underused by students. It is expensive to produce large numbers of handouts and often they go unread. Unless the information is vital and unobtainable in any other way, handouts are not the method of choice.

Exhibit 4–7 Instructions for CPR Participants

Special Instructions:

Individuals with any of the following conditions *will not be allowed* to participate in manikin testing and must be rescheduled for the class when the condition is no longer present.

1. Sore throat/cold
2. Other signs of infection (GI symptoms, rash, etc.)
3. Fever blister or other mouth lesion
4. Any open lesion on the hands
5. Recent back injury or other injury contraindicating manikin testing
6. Advanced pregnancy

Source: Education Department, Huntington Memorial Hospital, Pasadena, California. Reprinted with permission.

If you feel a handout is called for, following these guidelines will strengthen its use:

1. Edit content down to the minimum necessary.
2. Don't violate copyright laws—handing out multiple copies of journal articles or book chapters is not only lazy, it's dishonest.
3. Be sure the appearance of any handout is of the same high standard as the rest of your presentation.
4. Anything handed out before the class should relate to schedules or outlines; more detailed information will compete with the speaker.
5. If necessary, instruct participants to put the handouts down and direct their attention to the presentation.
6. If the handout is necessary for use in class, allow enough time for the slower readers to assimilate the information before proceeding.
7. Any handouts containing "nice-to-know" data should be available after class, not handed out during class.

Overhead Transparencies

The use of transparent acetate in conjunction with an overhead projector is widespread in hospital classrooms. Projectors are relatively inexpensive when compared with other hardware, and the transparencies are easy to make. They can be used in a lighted room with the instructor facing participants, thus maintaining interaction and feedback. Besides drawing or printing on the transparencies, you can duplicate pictures or print by loading the acetate sheets in a copying machine.

Through the use of colored pens or different shades of adhesive acetate, overlays and colorful displays can be created. Guidelines for using transparencies include:

1. Use black for the original.
2. Limit each transparency to a single point. An old rule used to be "six lines of copy, six words per line"—don't believe it. That much copy on a transparency is hard to read and boring.
3. Letters should be at least ¼ inch high. If you can read the original from ten feet away, you will have a readable transparency.
4. Place the projector so that keystoning, that stretched-out distortion when the angle to the screen is too sharp, is minimized.
5. Have an extra bulb on hand and know how to change it.
6. Leave each transparency on long enough for it to be read and for discussion of important points, but don't go on talking with the projector on once the points are made. Half the class will still be staring at the transparency or at the blank screen. Turn the machine off when you're not directly referring to the transparency.
7. Pencil lecture notes on the cardboard frames that hold the transparencies.

Bauman feels that the greatest misuse of transparencies occurs when they are employed as an "audio-visual blackboard" covered with words and more words.[27] Also, don't duplicate a page of print or endless typewritten lists. Use transparencies for visual impact and illustration or don't bother using them.

Chalkboards and Flipcharts

Both chalkboards and flipcharts are useful for noting discussion points or questions, listing important input from participants, and sketching explanatory drawings or diagrams. Chalkboards must be erased when filled up, which can result in information being lost. Flipchart pages can be torn off and taped around the walls so that input is saved for later referral. If you are preparing information before class to be presented later, turn the chalkboard around or cover the flipchart pages so that participants read the points only at the right time. Blank flipchart pages are best to cover the written ones, but be sure to allow *two* plain sheets between each printed one.

The same warning for handouts and transparencies holds true for chalkboards and flipcharts: don't cover them with a flood of words. Both chalkboard and flipchart can be hard to see from the back of the room, so go back there and check visibility before class begins. If you are using colored pens, stay away from light colors like yellow. Both chalkboard and flipchart are cost-effective methods, since chalkboards can be used and reused and flipcharts can be saved to repeat the same class again and again.

Slides

Slides project large visual images on the screen, and thus can be used for very big audiences. Because they are small, storage is easy. Keep them in trays or boxes to prevent soiling and loss. Using slides gives you flexibility because they can be added, deleted, or rearranged very quickly. When combined with an audiotape, a slide program can present an entire segment of information independently. Although fairly expensive because of development costs, slides can be used over and over again and give a polished and professional look with just a little extra effort.

Use the following guidelines when preparing slides:

1. Each slide should contain only one idea.
2. The best slides use pictures, symbols, or simple diagrams to make the point. Avoid long lists or complicated graphs and figures.
3. The proper aspect ratio (proportion of height to width) is 2:3 for slides.[28] As long as you keep the right height to width proportion, the size of the paper you do the artwork on won't matter.
4. Lettering should be large. Typewriter lettering is usually unreadable. Use press-on letters, print, or produce lettering with a machine such as a Kroy or Letteron.
5. When photographing for slides, best results are obtained with a 35 mm camera, but perfectly good slides can come from a simple Instamatic, using slide film and creativity.
6. Use blank slides at any pauses so you won't have to turn the machine on and off during class. Make these by cutting cardboard into slide-sized squares.
7. Always use a hand-held remote control to operate the projector. There is nothing more irritating than the incessant "Next slide, please."
8. Limit the number of slides to those absolutely necessary for highlighting important points. Too many slides will confuse rather than enlighten the learners.

Filmstrips

Filmstrips present explanations of procedures with great visual detail. The narration explains the visuals without the instructor having to speak, but at any time you can stop the presentation to elaborate a point or back up to review. The cost of the machine is usually little more than that of an overhead projector.

For most hospital instructors, the cost of making a filmstrip is prohibitive. For less cost and with less inconvenience a slide/sound show can be made. Thus most filmstrips are purchased from outside companies. The most obvious problems are lack of flexibility and difficulty in obtaining programs pertinent to your institution. A less obvious but frequently encountered problem with filmstrips is that many health care professionals dislike them. Whether they have found many filmstrips too basic or whether this attitude comes from overuse of filmstrips during basic preparatory programs, the fact remains that some of the orientees may automatically "turn off" when a filmstrip begins. Minimize this tendency by selecting excellent programs and giving a clear, objective-oriented introduction.

Films

Showing 16 mm films is an old tradition in hospital education. In the not-too-distant past the automatic response to any operational problem used to be "show them a film." However educationally unsound this was, the practice at least ensured that almost every hospital, no matter how small, owns a 16 mm film projector.

Unless you have a completely equipped studio with media professionals to man it, producing your own films is almost impossible. There are plenty of professional productions to choose from. If you are not already on mailing lists, get the names of several major media-producing companies from the purchasing department and send them your name and address. Film catalogs and announcements of new films will soon fill your mailbox.

In choosing a film there is one cardinal rule to follow: *always preview it before purchase*. That's the only way to be sure the film covers the right material and contributes to achieving your objectives. Don't get carried away by the description in the brochure; people are paid a lot of money to make every film sound like the answer to an instructor's prayers. See it yourself and ask these questions:

1. Does this film accomplish my previously written objectives? Don't purchase a film and try to work a class around it—make the film work for you.
2. Is the presentation effective? Could the same objectives be achieved by some cheaper and simpler method?
3. Is there anything in the film that might offend a member of the audience? Sometimes embarrassing or even prejudiced material slips into a film without its makers being aware of it. You must be aware.
4. Is the length right? Most films run from 20 to 30 minutes. Any longer than this and you risk losing the group's attention. On the other hand, a film that runs less than 15 minutes may not be giving you full value for your money.
5. How long will the film be usable? If the information will be outdated quickly, a less lasting (and less expensive) medium might be a better choice.

Unfortunately, the days of the free preview seem to be over. Almost all companies now charge a preview fee. This charge is applicable to the purchase price if you decide to buy the film, and if previewing prevents a single wrong purchase it pays for eight to sixteen previews in money saved. If the film is needed for only a short time (perhaps a subject for one group of orientees going to a specialty area), consider rental. The fee is usually moderate, but order well in advance to be sure of getting the date you want.

Once the film arrives, watch it several times so that you are thoroughly familiar with the content. Often the guide that comes with the film has discussion questions already prepared. If not, come up with your own. Always give participants something to do during the film. Know how to load and run the projector, and be prepared to cover the content if the film breaks or a fuse blows. After your introduction of the film and its key points, stay in the room. However tempting it may be to start the projector and leave after you have seen the film 20 times, you need to be present in case a bulb blows or something else goes wrong. Don't feel obligated to show the entire film. If only part of it is relevant, turn the projector off at that point and discuss what has been covered. Always end a film with a discussion of the key points and their applications.

The disadvantages of films don't outweigh their usefulness, but should be kept in mind. Films must be shown in darkness, which encourages inattention. Never show a film the first thing in the morning or right after lunch—half the class will fall asleep. Films cannot be updated or revised, so outdated information spoils their usefulness. If you have a film that provokes laughter because the actors are dressed in 1950 fashions and the equipment hasn't been used in your hospital for years, get rid of it. The information can be covered in ways that don't lose participants' attention and respect.

Videotape

Videotaping is coming into its own in hospitals. Although the initial cost of equipment is high, videotaping can be used in a number of ways. One way to get your budget request approved is to enlist physician support. Once the doctors have seen how easily surgery and other procedures can be taped, they usually become enthusiastic supporters.

Video can be used to show close-ups of small equipment or a roomful of people simulating a Code Blue response. At critical points the frame can be frozen to point out details, or the tape can be rewound to review a complicated procedure. Perhaps the greatest advantage to the use of videotape is its instant appeal to learners raised on television. This is a format everyone is familiar with—and likes.

Ideally, the hospital should have a media specialist, two video cameras, and an editor (a machine that edits shots from the two cameras into one finished tape). With this kind of media section, your productions can be professional—even marketable. If this is beyond your budget, one camera and a part-time consultant to teach taping techniques will yield effective presentations.

Videotaping is not something you learn from reading an instruction booklet. Hire a media specialist to teach you how to handle the equipment and produce tapes. One group of instructors thought they could do it all on their own. As they started taping their presentation on infection control they noticed that actor movement produced a blurred afterimage (a technical flaw that an expert could easily have corrected). To compensate for this, the actors tried to make no sudden moves. The result: a tape of instructors in isolation garb moving in slow motion. It was an expensive and embarrassing lesson.

When buying professional programs, check the format before you purchase. There are three formats available: ¾-inch, Beta, and VHS. None is compatible with the others. Most professional video programs for hospitals and other industries are in the ¾-inch format. The tapes are large and expensive, but can be reused again and again as you tape right over any program no longer needed. There are no developing costs and the tapes last a number of years.

When using videotaped procedures or dramatizations in class, the instructor must be aware of audience size. Only a small class—perhaps ten people—can see a 19-inch television screen well enough to make it useful as a teaching aid. If videotape is used for a larger group, more monitors must be provided, leading to potential problems with wiring and electrical overload. It's a good idea to have any setup checked for electrical safety.

Videotaping can be used live in class to record participants' actions and play them back for assessment and critique (as in mock patient interviews). However, this is very time consuming and thus not usually practical for orientation. Many people are uncomfortable being videotaped and may even refuse to participate, an additional problem to keep in mind.

Cost Effectiveness

There is no doubt about the suitability of audio-visual media for orientation programs. However, notice that effective audio-visual presentations require more effort to produce than simple lectures. The time involved includes planning, production, timing, and rehearsing both the educational approach and proper operation of equipment. Since orientees are used to television and motion pictures, they expect professional quality media, whether videotape, transparency, or handout. If your media production skills are limited to scrawling words on a chalkboard or flipchart, run—do not walk—to a workshop on the production and use of audio-visual materials.

CONCLUSION

The selection of teaching strategies must be based on the objectives the instructor wants the group to accomplish. Most instructors become comfortable with a few time-tested approaches and limit themselves to those familiar techniques. To increase teaching (and learning) effectiveness, instructors responsible for orientation should force themselves to try new methods and expand their teaching repertoires.

NOTES

1. Laura Mae Douglass and Em Olivia Bevis, *Nursing Leadership in Action* (St. Louis: C.V. Mosby Co., 1974), 31.

2. Malcolm S. Knowles, *The Modern Practice of Adult Education* (Chicago: Association Press, Follett Publishing Co., 1980), 47.

3. Ibid., 39.

4. Ascher J. Segall et al., *Systematic Course Design for the Health Care Fields* (New York: John Wiley and Sons, 1975), B–130.

5. Mary Louis Donaldson, "Instructional Media as a Teaching Stategy," *Nurse Educator* 4, no. 4 (July-August 1976): 18.

6. Agnes G. Rezler and Victor Rezmovic, "The Learning Preference Inventory," *Journal of Allied Health* 10, no. 2 (February 1981): 28.

7. Rebecca Partridge, "Learning Styles: A Review of Selected Models," *Journal of Nursing Education* 22, no. 6 (June 1983): 243.

8. Ibid., 244–245.

9. Ibid., 246.

10. David A. Kolb, *Learning Style Inventory* (Boston: McBer and Co., 1976), 7.

11. Rezler and Rezmovic, "The Learning Preference Inventory," 29.

12. Jerrold E. Kemp, *Instructional Design* (Belmont, Calif.: Lear Siegler/Fearon Publishers, 1971), 53.

13. Corinne B. Linton and James W. Truelove, *Hospital-Based Education* (New York: Arco Publishing, 1980), 72–73.

14. Marjorie Moore Cantor, "Education for Quality Care," *Journal of Nursing Administration* 5, no. 1 (January-February 1973): 13.

15. Jean Hayter, "How Good Is the Lecture as a Teaching Method?" *Nursing Outlook* 27, no. 4 (April 1979): 274.

16. W.A. Mambert, *Effective Presentations* (New York: John Wiley and Sons, 1976), 250.

17. Martin M. Broadwell, *The Supervisor as an Instructor: A Guide for Classroom Training,* 2d ed. (Reading, Mass.: Addison-Wesley Publishing Co., 1970), 79.

18. Rheba deTornyay and Martha A. Thompson, *Strategies for Teaching Nursing,* 2d ed. (New York: John Wiley and Sons, 1982), 94.

19. Karen Gahan Tarnow, "Working with Adult Learners," *Nurse Educator* 4, no. 5 (September-October 1979): 37.

20. deTornyay and Thompson, *Strategies,* 25.

21. *Training and Continuing Education: A Handbook for Health Care Institutions* (Chicago: Hospital Research and Educational Trust, 1970), 36–1.

22. Carolyn Chambers Clark, "Simulation Gaming: A New Teaching Strategy in Nursing Education," *Nurse Educator* 1, no. 4 (November-December 1976): 76.

23. Linda Standke, "Using Games To Help Meet Your Objectives," *TRAINING* 32, no. 12 (December 1978): 76.

24. Patricia A. McLagan, *Helping Others Learn: Designing Programs for Adults* (Reading, Mass.: Addison-Wesley Publishing Co., 1978), 35.

25. Mambert, *Effective Presentations,* 220.

26. Neil F. Duane, "An Audiovisual Overview," *Nurse Educator* 4, no. 4 (July-August 1979): 7.

27. Karen Bauman and Alice Kirkman Kunka, "Overhead Transparencies: The Overlooked Medium," *Nurse Educator* 4, no. 4 (July-August 1979): 21.

28. Claudia Schmalenberg, "Making and Using Slides," *Nurse Educator* 4, no. 4 (July-August 1979): 12.

Part II

Orientation of Allied Employees

Chapter 5

New Employee Orientation

New employee orientation refers to the time set aside to orient all new employees, regardless of department, job description, and rank, to the hospital system. The time allotted can run from a few minutes to two full days, and the content varies from hospital to hospital, but the basic principle remains the same: *everyone* attends.

As we saw in Chapter 1, in the past many hospitals provided orientation only for nurses, ignoring new employees from the allied departments. This discrimination not only caused problems from a labor relations standpoint but resulted in serious operating difficulties later on, as the inadequately oriented people spread through the organization.

Gillies states unequivocably: ''General indoctrination should be standardized for all employees of the institution."[1] The two arguments against this are that it costs too much and that the employees are needed in their departments immediately. Neither is defensible. The costs of new employee orientation are minimal compared with the costs of mistakes and turnover caused by inadequate orientation. As for needing an employee instantly, it is hard to believe that one day makes that much difference after a department has done without the person throughout the recruiting and hiring period. Nursing managers will be glad to describe the benefits of waiting for an oriented employee; they have been doing it for years.

People entering a new job situation are anxious and vulnerable, but this very anxiety heightens their motivation to learn. New employees want to like the organization and their roles in it. If the hospital uses this predisposition to best advantage, employees can be socialized into the system as productive, satisfied workers

TIMING OF HOSPITALWIDE ORIENTATION

Orientation should take place during the first week of employment, preferably the very first day, if the new employee is to feel at home in the hospital and identify with its goals. The employee needs information about the organization and the different roles within the system immediately. After workers have joined their departments they receive input from co-workers about policies and procedures that may be distorted by misunderstanding or personal feelings. Tobin feels that one of the major objectives of an orientation program is to reduce and control the number of sources from which new employees receive information.[2]

Another consideration developed by Gillies is that new employees are especially susceptible to the influence of authority figures when first entering the institution.[3] This is due to lack of information about the situation as well as anxiety. If the new employees' first exposure to policies and benefits is given in an organized, positive fashion by a credible, well-informed hospital representative, identification with the organization is likely to occur. Later, when new employees are more familiar with the work situation, acceptance may not be so automatic.

SCHEDULING

Upon hire employees should be informed about the orientation program. Informing them does not mean saying "Be in the education department at 8:00 Monday." It involves giving them a class schedule and explaining how new employee orientation will help them adjust to their new environment. The personnel department has the responsibility for doing this, through recruiters or their secretaries who handle the after-hire paperwork.

One strategy that has been found to enhance employee support of the institution is the letter of welcome.[4] This should come from the hospital administrator. Mailed to the new employee's home, it welcomes the new person to the hospital and offers best wishes for success in the new job role. Exhibit 5–1 shows an example of a letter of welcome. Note how this first after-hire communication refers to the new employee's department and maintains a warm tone.

A last important facet of scheduling orientation involves communication between Personnel and the people responsible for orientation—the managers and instructors. Managers have the overall responsibility for orienting their employees. What part of orientation is handled by the individual manager and what is delegated to others depends on hospital policy and individual employee needs, but the manager is the person with ultimate accountability. After the decision to hire has been made and a start date set, inform the employee's manager about orientation. When is the new person scheduled to begin? How long will classes last? This is usually standardized, but if a long time has passed since the last new hire the manager may have forgotten the timing of the orientation process.

The education department should administer what Otto calls "common denominator training."[5] This is any program given to large numbers of employees and repeated with reasonable frequency. New employee orientation certainly fits

Exhibit 5–1 Letter of Welcome

Dear

Welcome to the staff of Hometown General Hospital. Your knowledge and experience will be invaluable to the ______________________________

Department and to our institution. As you become familiar with the hospital and your department, we invite you to participate in the discussion and decision making involved in providing the best care for our patients.

Your orientation is planned to begin on ______________________________. This initial period of employment is designed to help you learn how things work and where you fit into the system and your work group. We hope you will find this process informative and helpful as you become part of our team. If you have any questions or concerns about your role or the hospital, please ask your manager right away.

Again, welcome to our hospital. We hope to have a long and fulfilling partnership with you. Good luck in reaching your goals.

Sincerely,

John Q. Administrator
Chief Executive Officer

this category. When an employee is hired, Personnel notifies Education and the new person is added to the next program. The minimum information needed is name, department, position, and date of starting employment. Even more helpful is additional data about past work experience. Someone who has just moved into the area can benefit from maps, restaurant guides, and other welcoming paraphernalia that the education department has available.

In some hospitals orientation takes place whenever a new person is hired. If the employee wants to begin working on a Wednesday, someone from Education is assigned to orient them that Wednesday. Another new person may begin the next day, and so on. This practice wastes time and money and results in poor quality orientation. Dates for new employee orientation should be set in advance. Once the system is established, the dates are automatically self-perpetuating. How often induction is scheduled depends on the hospital and the number of new hires. The most frequent schedule seems to be twice a month, with some hospitals opting for once a month and others every two weeks. Once a week does not seem to be a practice, though such a system is certainly possible.

Whatever the scheduling decided on, new people should be hired with the orientation dates in mind. Instead of starting them on Wednesday, schedule the first day of employment for the next Monday when new employee orientation is given. No well-managed department should need help so desperately that a few days wait is intolerable. Starting new employees only on certain set dates provides time for reference checks and makes orientation an organized process, where the all-important first impression is of smooth efficiency. Contrast that with the harried, almost frantic impression made on new employees when a hospital is willing to start them any day, any time. People like structure, especially in institutions they've decided to join.

PROGRAM CONTENT

Hospitalwide orientation should provide new employees with information about three basic subjects:

1. The organization as a whole and as a number of departments working together to accomplish a mission.
2. The ground rules for working in the organization.
3. The advantages of working for the organization.[6]

Within these broad categories are numerous possible subjects.

What is required by law to be presented in new employee orientation? Besides requiring that certain departments be involved in the orientation and training of new employees, JCAH makes several specific statements regarding orientation content. For instance, "The governing body, through the chief executive officer, shall ensure that written personnel policies and practices that adequately support optimal achievable patient care are established and maintained. The policies shall be made available to all employees and shall be discussed with each new employee."[7] Other JCAH requirements include information on fires, internal and external disasters, safety (particularly electrical safety), infection control, and CPR.

How this required information is presented depends on the hospital and the instructor. Electrical safety could be covered by passing around a handout, or it could be the subject of an entire class. Personnel policies may be discussed in new employee orientation, covered in detail by managers of the individual departments, or presented in written form in an employee handbook. Fire safety, infection control, disasters—these subjects may be addressed by lecture, film, handouts, games, and all the other teaching strategies discussed in Chapter 4.

Personnel category influences the depth and detail of presentation. A nurse would need to know more about infection control than an accountant; that much is obvious. But how much does a laundry worker need to know about the subject? What about a dietary worker? This wide range of need suggests that a general introduction to the subject be given during new employee orientation and the specifics be covered during department/unit orientation.

Besides reading through the JCAH manual for specific guidelines for orientation content, be sure to check state laws (such as California's Title 22) for required information. Individual hospitals also set policies on what should be covered, particularly in regard to information on body mechanics, confidentiality and other legal aspects of care, and employee certification in CPR. Exhibit 5–2 is a list of topics covered in a typical hospitalwide orientation program. This particular course is one and one-half days long.

To avoid overloading new employees with details they won't remember, take a look at how many employees are likely to need each item of information and how soon they will need it. Knowles feels that an orientation program should not start with the history and philosophy of the organization, but rather with real-life concerns of new workers: Where will I be working? What will be expected of me? How do people dress here? To whom can I go for help?[8] This doesn't mean that the history and philosophy won't be covered—merely that perhaps it shouldn't be covered *first*. Take a look at the organization of the content. Is it logically arranged? What areas are most interesting? You may feel that the history and

---

Exhibit 5–2 New Employee Orientation Topics

Getting to know you
History of the hospital
Administrative structure
Hospital department presentation
Personnel services
Policies/Benefits
Hospital floor plan
Computer system
Education department
Body mechanics
Infection control
Disaster plan
Notification reporting system
Accident reporting system
Electrical safety
Fire safety
Security

Source: Education Department, Huntington Memorial Hospital, Pasadena, California. Reprinted with permission.

philosophy of the hospital is a nice lead-in to a discussion of the employee's role in the organization or that a slide/sound presentation on the subject would go best after the break. Arrange the content in the way that seems most helpful, with more enjoyable activities interspersed throughout the dry areas of necessary content.

To help with this process, Shea suggests some questions the instructor can ask:

1. What specific things will the person need to know about the new environment to be comfortable, safe, and well oriented? (Restrooms, transportation, food, etc.)
2. What important impressions do I want to make on that first day? (This question can also be, "If I were a new employee, what would be important for me to know?")
3. What *key* policies and procedures must this employee know on the first day so mistakes won't be made on the second?
4. What positive experience can I provide for the new person to talk about to the "folks at home"?[9]

There will never be enough time for all the information you would like to cover, but for the sake of cost control as well as for the new employees, who are anxious to get to their jobs, new employee orientation should be limited to no longer than two days. Many fine programs are one day in length.

If managers feel strongly that new employees should be introduced to their departments on the first day, a split program might be used, with two half days or a longer first day and shorter second one. Exhibit 5–3 shows a ten-hour program split into two days. The course covers all required information, including fire and electrical safety and infection control. The only information not provided is CPR. It cannot be stressed too strongly that CPR training should be provided in a separate class. Teaching resuscitation skills properly requires at least four hours in order to allow adequate time for manikin practice.

CONDUCTING NEW EMPLOYEE ORIENTATION

Guest Speakers

After reserving a room, the instructor must arrange for speakers. Although the entire program can be presented by one person, there are several arguments against this. First, listening to the sound of the same voice for a long period can have a soporific effect. Even with different teaching strategies and media, a single instructor is not as interesting as a variety of people. Second, conducting new employee orientation is exhausting work if done correctly, with a great deal of individualized attention. And third, valuable socialization can occur from a wise choice of speakers. The speaker with the greatest impact is the hospital admin-

Exhibit 5–3 New Employee Orientation Course Description

Monday	
Getting to Know You	Group warm-up activity
History of the Hospital	Orientation instructor
Organizational Structure	Orientation instructor
Hospital Departments and Roles	Orientation instructor
(Break)	
Welcome from Administration	Hospital administrator
Personnel Services	Personnel director
Policies and Benefits	Employee representative
Hospital Floor Plan	Orientation instructor
(Lunch)	
Computer System	Computer services
(All participants report to their departments.)	
Thursday	
Education Department	Director of Education
Electrical Safety/Fire Safety	Security department
Safety and Security Programs	Security department
(Break)	
Accident/Incident Reporting	Orientation instructor
Overview of Disaster Plan	Orientation instructor
Body Mechanics	Orientation instructor
Infection Control	Nurse epidemiologist
Evaluation of Program	Group
(All participants return to assigned area after lunch.)	

istrator. By devoting a short amount of time every two weeks or so, the administrator initiates a positive relationship between new employees and the organization. Studies show that a feeling of belonging is related to seeing and talking to VIPs, even if only once.[10]

Other speakers might include a personnel representative to present highlights of employee benefits, the nurse epidemiologist to talk about infection control, or a biomedical engineer to discuss electrical safety. Besides making sure that having these speakers will contribute to achieving your objectives, you may want to follow these guidelines for choosing guests:

1. The speaker should be a recognized expert in whatever is being discussed.
2. Presentations should hold interest, which requires the ability to relate to orientees and entails more than just a lively speaking style.

3. Any speakers selected must be able to stay within set time limits. A speaker who consistently runs overtime, wrecking your carefully orchestrated schedule, must be replaced. (If the administrator is the offender, change the schedule.)

Avoid sensory overload and confusion by controlling the number of presenters. For a full-day program, four guest speakers are plenty, especially if films or videotapes are used during the day.

After arranging when and where each speaker will present, give them the objectives for their presentations. Stress that these objectives describe what the orientees should be able to do after listening to the talk. Time guidelines should be discussed, along with the fact that you will signal when the time is up. A few days before the first few orientations that a speaker will be appearing in, send a reminder note with date, place, and time. And occasionally show your appreciation by having a luncheon for your speakers and sending them periodic thank-you cards.

Packets

Once speakers have been contacted and provided with objectives and time limits, the instructor must tackle the problem of packets. What handouts and forms will be included in the packet that the new employees receive as they enter the classroom? Avoid overwhelming them with printed material. If too many pages pile up, too few will be read. A workable list of handouts might include:

1. Schedule for the program with timing and breaks
2. Objectives for the program
3. Map of the hospital
4. Organization chart (with key names included)
5. List of patients' rights
6. Copy of employee handbook
7. Evaluation form

Keep aside handouts pertaining to specific topics, such as Infection Control or Fire Safety, and pass them out during that segment of the program. This increases their impact and reduces the bombardment of paper that the new employee faces early on the first day. Also try to allow time *in class* for reading everything handed out. For instance, go over the schedule and objectives verbally with the participants, explaining them in greater detail and encouraging questions. Review "Patients' Rights" using audio-visual highlights and discussing the implications this document has for employees. The only exception to this rule might be the employee handbook if it is lengthy. But at least go over the contents and have the group pick it up and leaf through it during class. By stressing the importance of the information in the handbook and by getting the participants used to handling it, you may increase the likelihood of its being read.

Some instructors might question the inclusion of the evaluation form. Why is it placed in the initial packet rather than handed out at the end of the program? Exhibit 5–4 shows a sample form for evaluation of new employee orientation. If such a form is given to the participants at the beginning of class and its purpose explained, notes can be made on it as class progresses. This prevents a frantic last-minute scramble to remember all the different presentations or, even worse, no responses at all. Few people are willing to write helpful comments when two minutes remain and the instructor announces brightly "Please fill out those evaluation forms before you leave."

Exhibit 5–4 New Employee Orientation Evaluation Form

The Education Department has a sincere desire to continue building our effectiveness in assisting new employees through the orientation process. One of the ways we hope to meet this challenge is through feedback from our participants. As educators we learn not only from our accomplishments but also from our mistakes.

Please take a moment to assist us in making this program better by sharing your thoughts and suggestions. You may wish to consider the following aspects in the evaluation of the individual speakers and presentations:

- Extent to which the presentation maintained my interest
- Presenter's methods of delivery (diction, eye contact, enthusiasm, response to questions, rapport, explanation, etc.)
- Organization of content
- Value to new employee

Partners in Tradition (film)

Administrative structure

Hospital department presentation

Administrative welcome

Personnel services

Policies and benefits

C.A.R.E.S. presentation

Source: Education Department, Huntington Memorial Hospital, Pasadena, California. Reprinted with permission.

The Program

First impressions influence the whole course of orientation, and ultimately the entire adjustment of new employees to the new work setting. In order to control those vital first impressions, the instructor should arrive at the class site early and be sure everything is set up—seating, equipment, films, packets, etc. Refreshments should be available at the beginning of the program. If you make people wait until the break for their coffee, they will have trouble concentrating on the information presented.

Have a sign-in table at the door to welcome each new employee. If possible, a colleague should sit there, greeting each participant and assisting with packets and name cards. If no one is available, a sign such as the one in Exhibit 5–5 can be placed by the table. The lead instructor should not be tied down at the table; it is important to circulate around the room and talk with orientees. Never forget one

---

Exhibit 5–5 Sign Greeting Orientees

WELCOME TO NEW EMPLOYEE ORIENTATION!!

PLEASE:

1. USING THE MAGIC MARKER, PRINT YOUR FIRST NAME AND YOUR DEPARTMENT ON THE LARGE FOLDED CARD AND KEEP IT WITH YOU. EXAMPLE:

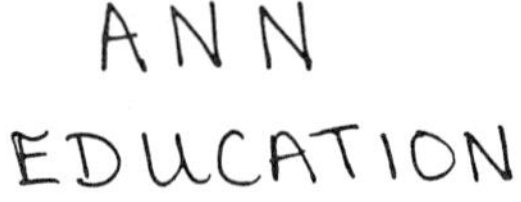

2. PRINT YOUR FIRST AND LAST NAMES ON A BADGE AND PUT IT ON:

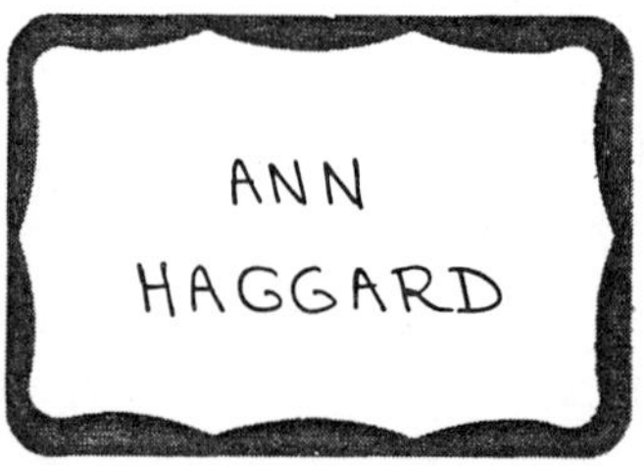

3. SIGN YOUR NAME AND DEPARTMENT ON THE ROLL SHEET.

4. TAKE A TAN FOLDER AND FIND A SEAT (COFFEE, TEA, HOT CHOCOLATE, AND DECAFFEINATED COFFEE ARE TO YOUR LEFT).

vital fact: you are the host or hostess of new employee orientation. Concentrate on welcoming your guests and making them feel at home.

Begin within five minutes of the stated starting time, whether everyone is there or not. Not only is it unfair to punish the people who came on time by making them wait but if you get behind now, you'll never catch up. To be sure no important content is missed by latecomers, open with a warm-up exercise. At this point the participants are a roomful of strangers, waiting to hear another stranger speak to them. Warm-up exercises change this anxious atmosphere to one of camaraderie.

Ricks feels that the instructor's initial task should be to bring people to the point where:

1. They can work comfortably together in an unfamiliar environment.
2. They will draw freely on the special resources the instructor provides.
3. They have set some positive goals to achieve.[11]

There are many ways to accomplish this. After introducing yourself and welcoming everyone to the program and to the institution, get people moving. Divide the group into subgroups of five or six members and give them some task to do; finding out about one another in order to introduce someone to the total group is always a good one. Move around the room while this is going on and address each group separately. Your goal with this exercise is to set up social units within which an individual can exert influence.[12] Throughout the day, people will speak up more because they feel supported by their "team."

Once this rapport is established, the content can be presented to a much more open group. The role of the instructor throughout the day is multifaceted—you must maintain the friendly atmosphere, be sure the guest speakers show up and leave on time, answer questions, and tend to housekeeping details such as coffee refills. One tricky duty is to defuse potentially volatile situations. Perhaps one orientee becomes upset over something during the discussion of benefits; although this person has a right to be upset, the incident must not be allowed to disrupt the presentation for the rest of the participants. You may have to take the angry employee from the room and speak privately, perhaps suggesting a discussion with the personnel department or the individual's manager. Whatever happens, you must *cope*.

Keep the methods of presentation as varied and interesting as you can. Using principles from Chapter 4, select teaching strategies most conducive to accomplishing the established objectives. If you want orientees to recognize the top administrators, pictures of these key people are needed, either as slides or on a large poster. Excellent films on fire and electrical safety are available, or a hospital-specific video program could be made. When covering benefits or regulations, the presentation should be limited to highlights only. Don't expect orientees to remember the details—they're too overloaded with information. Refer them to the employee handbook for later study.

Most experts recommend that the new employees be given a hospital tour on the first day.[13] Ideally this should be a live, walking tour, but for very large groups it could be on film. A large group could also be split up and taken around the hospital in small groups, but if this is done, be very careful about who conducts these subgroups. During a tour of the facility the person leading the group can make seemingly unimportant comments that have tremendous impact on the new employees. An offhand murmur of "And over here is where Administration has breakfast meetings—that's all they ever seem to do, ha, ha," can establish an indelible attitude toward Administration. Control the information received by conducting tours yourself or trusting subgroups only to colleagues you know will present a positive and vital image of the hospital. Tours are not a task to be left to unknown volunteers.

Many organizations provide a free lunch to new employees on the first day. If this can be done, arrange to make the luncheon another step toward socializing orientees into the system. Rather than handing out lunch tickets and turning the group loose in the cafeteria, have Food Service set up a simple buffet. Invite the manager and/or mentor of each new employee to this luncheon. After getting their food, the orientees and guests can sit down and get to know one another in a relaxed, nonwork situation.

CONCLUSION

At the end of new employee orientation, the orientees should leave the room feeling more familiar and at ease with their new environment. Your efforts at building rapport and imparting information begin with scheduling orientation and planning the content, progress through preparing speakers and providing handout information, and culminate in a productive classroom experience.

The next chapter examines department orientation, the follow-up to new employee orientation. It is within the individual departments that orientees become functioning staff members, so what happens there will ultimately affect an orientee's career and a hospital's bottom line. Chapter 6 presents guidelines for that all-important process.

NOTES

1. Dee Ann Gillies, *Nursing Management: A Systems Approach* (Philadelphia: W.B. Saunders Co., 1982), 205.
2. Helen M. Tobin, Pat S. Yoder-Wise, and Peggy K. Hull, *The Process of Staff Development: Components for Change*, 2d ed. (St. Louis: C.V. Mosby Co., 1979), 159.
3. Gillies, *Nursing Management*, 206–207.

4. Julius Yourman, "Orientation of New Employees," in *Improving the Effectiveness of Hospital Management,* ed. Addison C. Bennett (New York: Metromedia Analearn, 1972), 252.

5. Calvin P. Otto and Rollin O. Glaser, *The Management of Training* (Reading, Mass.: Addison-Wesley Publishing Co., 1970), 345.

6. Ibid., 343.

7. *Accreditation Manual for Hospitals, 1983 Edition* (Chicago: Joint Commission on Accreditation of Hospitals, 1983), 80–81.

8. Malcolm S. Knowles, *The Modern Practice of Adult Education* (Chicago: Association Press, Follett Publishing Co., 1980), 53.

9. Gordon F. Shea, "Supervising New Employees," *Training and Development Journal* 36, no. 1 (January 1982): 52.

10. Yourman, "Orientation of New Employees," 252.

11. Don M. Ricks, "Making the Most of the First 20 Minutes of Your Training," in *Adult Learning in Your Classroom,* ed. Philip G. Jones (Minneapolis: Lakewood Publications, 1982), 14.

12. Ibid., 59.

13. Yourman, "Orientation of New Employees," 252.

Chapter 6

Department Orientation

What happens to new employees after they leave new employee orientation? Often they are left to sink or swim on their own, and all too many sink. Day-to-day pressures and crises force departments to rush orientees into unfamiliar roles, figuring that full orientation can wait until the crunch is over. Aside from the fact that another crisis usually follows hard after the current one, this practice is short-sighted for a number of reasons. A well-planned orientation can prevent mistakes and accidents, increase productivity, and decrease turnover, as we have noted. One study found that turnover was 491 percent higher among employees who had been on the job less than a year, compared with those who remained for a longer period of time.[1] Once department heads ponder that figure, they will realize that haphazard orientation is too expensive a practice to follow.

Beginnings are important. The very early hours and days in a new work environment are critical to the motivation, attitude, and behavior of a new employee.[2] Allowing orientees to learn by trial and error—and practice mistakes until they become habits—broadcasts an unmistakable message of indifference. On the other hand, conducting an effective orientation for new people demonstrates to all employees that the hospital cares about its workers. The institution may also discover serendipitous benefits: higher productivity, better organization, and more efficiency.

COORDINATING DEPARTMENT ORIENTATION

In some hospitals the allied educators in the education department coordinate department orientation; in others it is solely the job of the department head and supervisors. Regardless of how your particular system is organized, a hospital's professional educators owe it to the institution and the new employees to help line managers develop the best possible department orientation programs.

Involving the allied departments in this or any task is not easy. You are dealing with many different disciplines, all with different priorities and values. If an educational problem arises with nursing personnel, the instructor contacts the director of nursing, who can call all head nurses together to work on a solution. Allied departments repcrt to different administrators, so there is almost never an occasion when all allied department heads are together. This means that your communication must be conducted by memo and one-on-one conferences.

One way to involve the allied departments is through an education advisory committee similar to the one discussed in Chapter 2 as a needs assessment tool. In some hospitals there is a hospitalwide advisory committee that addresses educational issues affecting all employees and a separate allied advisory committee concerned only with non-nursing areas. If departments have an employee responsible for education—a senior employee who orients and trains all workers in the department—those allied educators would be ideal for committee membership. Some hospitals require that allied department heads serve on the committee. In others membership is voluntary.

However the committee is organized, its aim remains the same: to ensure consistency and quality for all allied education programs, including orientation. Members can draw up an overall plan for department orientation, not dictating content, which will differ from area to area, but providing structure and guidance in the orientation process.

If your hospital has no education advisory committee, the best thing to do is organize one, but that can take time. In the meantime, you will have to work with individual department heads. Your aim is to help them increase their department's productivity and decrease turnover by organizing the orientation process. Keep that firmly in mind as you approach each manager. Don't come on as the all-knowing expert here to bail them out of the mess of their poorly designed program; that's a quick way to land back in your office wondering why no one listens to you. You are a staff expert assigned to serve as a resource for line managers—that is the real job of a hospital educator. You know "tricks of the trade" that will help the department heads develop orientation programs that *work*. Present your ideas in a businesslike manner, stressing bottom-line considerations.

Most managers accept the concept of an organized orientation program with no problems. What they worry about is the time involved in implementing comprehensive orientation. Use facts and figures to convince them that well-run orientation will be cheaper and easier for everyone concerned. Then make suggestions streamlining orientation for each department, working with the department head and any designated department instructors.

PLANNING DEPARTMENT ORIENTATION

According to Gillies the purpose of orientation is "to make the new employee feel wanted, needed, and expected by coworkers and supervisors and to make him believe his presence is required for realization of organizational goals."[3] Keeping that overall purpose in mind helps target planning and development of department orientation. If the department can socialize new employees into the system effectively, the bottom-line goals of reducing turnover, establishing good work habits, and increasing productivity should automatically result.

Since department managers are ultimately responsible for orienting new employees, selection of content and its delivery are up to them. But as managers work through this process, remind them to consult with their employees. The line workers who actually do the work are the best source of information on what a new person needs to learn.

Defining Objectives

Before objectives can be developed, the manager must define the job responsibilities. This starts with a review of the job description. Read through this list of duties as if you were the orientee. What is missing? Why do these tasks need to be performed? What makes this job different from similar positions in other institutions? One reading is enough to make it clear that the job description is only the beginning.

Does the department have written performance standards? A performance standard is a statement that completes this sentence for each major duty or task: "Performance is satisfactory when . . ."[4] Exhibit 6–1 is an example of a job description with accompanying standards, in this case for an allied instructor in an education department. Guide managers through the development of such standards by showing examples and having them write standards for their own positions. This experience demonstrates that standards must be developed with input from workers currently performing the jobs since only they know if the performance standards are realistic or not.

The written performance standards automatically supply objective, measurable criteria for evaluating performance. When reviewing the job description and standards with an orientee, the manager can make clear exactly how performance will be measured and pay raises awarded, preventing later misunderstandings.

The final step before actually developing objectives consists of reviewing the hospital and department goals and objectives for the year. These must be made clear to new employees so that they grasp the department's relationship to other departments and to the organization as a whole. The sooner orientees realize that their jobs are part of an overall effort to deliver quality health care, the sooner they will develop a spirit of camaraderie and teamwork.

Exhibit 6–1 Job Description with Standards

DEPARTMENT: Education	JOB CODE: 123
JOB TITLE: Allied Health Instructor	DATE REVIEWED: 10/83

SUMMARY OF DUTIES:
Responsible for designing, implementing, and facilitating new and continuing education programs and orientation for allied health personnel, under the direction of the Human Resources Development Manager.

RESPONSIBILITIES	STANDARDS
1.0 EDUCATION	
1.1 Plans, arranges, coordinates, and implements new employee orientation and safety programs.	Sends schedule of orientation dates to Personnel each 6 months. Evaluates and updates program on a regular basis. Ensures presence of guest instructors. Utilizes a variety of instructional methods and principles of adult education.
1.2 Plans, arranges, coordinates, and implements a program of staff development and continuing education for allied health personnel.	Programs should be based on needs assessment and performance data. Utilizes a variety of instructional methods and principles of adult education. Uses a variety of publicity techniques to encourage attendance. Evaluates programs. Ensures compliance with laws and regulations.
2.0 EDUCATION RESOURCE	
2.1 Serves as an education resource for allied departments.	Participates in annual needs assessment. Meets with individual members of allied departments to work on projects on request. Works closely with department instructors. Participates in monthly meeting with nursing department.
3.0 BUDGET/RECORD KEEPING	
3.1 Responsible for course documentation.	Ensures compliance with JCAH, Title 22, and BRN. Accurate and timely.

Exhibit 6–1 continued

DEPARTMENT: Education	JOB CODE: 123
JOB TITLE: Allied Health Instructor	
PAGE 2	
3.2 Maintains accurate records of course hours, attendance, and cost.	Submits accurate course report within 4 days after the class. Submits accurate monthly report no later than the third of the following month.
3.3 Evaluates new instructional materials for possible purchase.	Considers appropriateness of format, usage, and factors of cost containment.
3.4 Assists in preparation of department budget and in planning resources and facilities needed to perform responsibilities.	Assesses needed operating material for budget year. Shows attitude of cost consciousness by setting priorities in desired material. Operates within approved budget.
4.0 PROFESSIONAL	
4.1 Serves as a committee member on various hospital committees.	Represents education and the patient in the decision-making aspect of committees. Attends the meetings that have direct relevance to the position. Communicates information to appropriate department members. Evaluates current situation and proposes changes as indicated.
4.2 Keeps abreast of new theories and techniques in the allied health field and education.	Attends two conferences per year and keeps up to date by reading professional journals.
4.3 Assists in the development of philosophy, objectives, policies, and procedures for the education department.	Prepares well-written proposals when needed. Continuously re-evaluates current policies and procedures and recommends appropriate changes.
4.4 Functions effectively as a member of the education team.	Relates well to coworkers and hospital staff. Willingly offers assistance to staff where needed without being requested to do so.

Source: Joyce Johnson, Director of Education, Huntington Memorial Hospital, Pasadena, California. Reprinted with permission.

Writing orientation objectives for the department is really a two-part process. First, overall objectives must be established: what should *every* department employee learn during orientation? Exhibit 6–2 is an example of overall objectives for a department. Note that the objectives are written from an action viewpoint—what employees should be able to *do*. Review Chapter 3 for information on how to develop instructional objectives as managers are guided through this step.

Once department objectives are written, individual objectives should be prepared for each orientee. These objectives are based on the needs of the person in light of his or her background and experience and the requirements of the job. They should be developed with the new person after a review of the job description, performance standards, and department objectives. What must be learned during orientation (over and above the overall department orientation objectives)? The list will be different for each employee and need not be elaborate. Exhibit 6–3 is an example of individual objectives. (Note the suggestions for how they can be accomplished). After agreement is reached on these objectives, the manager and orientee each receive a copy, which serves as a guide for that person's orientation within the department.

Developing the Orientation Plan

Once objectives have been chosen, the information must be organized in a logical manner. One way to do this is to list general headings with pertinent information included under each heading (see Exhibit 6–4). By adding and

Exhibit 6–2 Overall Department Objectives

By the end of the orientation program, the new pharmacy employee should be able to:

1. Badge in and out correctly.
2. Use phones correctly and locate phone directory.
3. Describe job functions and the organization of the department.
4. Locate and use the policy and procedure manual.
5. Locate various pharmacy areas, including the IV area.
6. Describe the procedure to be followed if an employee is injured on the job.
7. Describe the pharmacy security system and the role of each pharmacy employee in maintaining it.
8. List the drugs and requisitions that can be delivered via the pneumatic tube system.
9. List the dates and locations of department meetings.
10. Locate all pharmacy stock.
11. Locate all pharmacy labels and forms.
12. Deliver ordered drugs to the correct satellite pharmacy within 15 minutes or less.

Exhibit 6–3 Individual Employee Objectives for a Clinical Laboratory Orientee

During the first three months, the employee will:

1. Develop a working knowledge of the computerized reporting system so that reports are accurate and delivered no later than 15 minutes after test completion.
2. Perform all operations in the biochemistry section.
3. Observe activities in the other sections in order to begin training in different areas at a date to be selected later.
4. Attend the inservice series "Interpretation of Laboratory Results" and work with the instructors, with the goal of teaching the section on biochemistry tests within six months.

Exhibit 6–4 General Headings for Department Orientation

Organization
- Goals and objectives
- Hospital philosophy
- Department philosophy
- Organization charts (administrative and department)
- Specific job description (roles, responsibilities, pay, work schedule, performance evaluations)
- Preceptor orientation (introduce preceptor)

Policies and procedures
- Hospital policy book
- Department policy and procedure manual
- Department rules and regulations
- Employee handbook
- General manuals (infection control, fire safety, disaster)
- Non-hospital manuals (JCAH, Title 22)

Physical facility
- Tour of department/work area
- Tour of hospital and key departments
- Location of equipment and supplies

Personnel
- Introduction to department employees
- Introduction to key employees from other departments

deleting subheadings and rearranging the order of priority, the manager identifies just what must be covered.

Now decisions must be made about the order and intensity of presentation. Beware of overwhelming orientees with information on the first day in the department. Belker found that many new employees go home from their first day on the job with a bad headache or other physical symptoms as a result of nervous tension.[5] Use the first day to introduce the orientee to the work group and the environment in a low-key, relaxed manner. Naturally, some information will be covered, but it should relate to general policies and personnel details rather than core data about the job. Review what was covered in new employee orientation and answer questions that have arisen overnight. Actual job training should definitely not begin the first day. Exhibit 6–5 shows a typical department orientation schedule. Notice that job training does not begin until the third day in the department.

Exhibit 6–5 Typical Department Orientation Schedule

First Day

1. Questions and comments about new employee orientation
2. Schedule and activities
3. Introduction of preceptor
4. Distribution of information (job description, organization chart, computer cards, uniform and name tags, etc.)
5. Tour of department and introduction of personnel
6. Review of hospital policy and procedure manuals
7. Review of department policy and procedure manuals
8. Questions and answers

Second Day

1. Review of information covered yesterday
2. Dress code
3. Department meeting schedule
4. Non-smoking policy
5. Fire safety manuals and procedures
6. Infection control procedures
7. Personal phone calls and personal belongings
8. Scheduling (including vacation policy)
9. Reporting sick and overtime
10. Performance evaluations
11. Questions and answers

Preparing the Work Group

Announce the hiring of a new employee as soon as the decision is made, so co-workers have a chance to get used to the idea before the orientee arrives. If appropriate, send a memo about the new person to all departments. A few days before the first day of induction, meet with the work group to give them background information about the new employee, an orientation schedule, and discuss how they can help their new co-worker feel welcome. Be sure someone is appointed to take the orientee along on lunch and breaks.

This preparation of department members takes little time but reaps great benefits. Employees tend to form a positive mind set toward new people when they are involved in planning the welcome. And orientees appreciate that welcome. There is nothing more devastating for a new employee than to arrive at a new department and find that he or she is not expected. "Who are you—I don't know anything about a new employee." That kind of welcome sets a negative tone that permeates the whole employment.

Preparing the Preceptor

Many departments use experienced employees as preceptors for new people. The assigned worker teaches the orientee not only job skills but how to get along in the system. Being clued in to the values and mores of the work group and hospital is invaluable to new workers. Some managers wish to do all training personally, and this approach is fine if the manager has the time to orient all new employees. For most people, delegation to a qualified preceptor is a must.

Choosing preceptors is a delicate task. Occasionally, organizations let the person leaving the job train the replacement. Unless the incumbent is being promoted for outstanding work, this may not be a good idea. Aside from the risk of deliberate misinformation being given by a bitter employee, the chances of the orientee receiving thorough instruction are slim. Even if orientation is done by employees who are not terminating, training may be incomplete. If the designated person doesn't know how to train, the new employee will probably not learn the job correctly. Some departments prepare a senior employee as a trainer, sending an excellent worker to classes on teaching techniques and principles of education.

Before starting a new employee, meet with the preceptor to outline the course of orientation and how it is to be handled. This discussion should take place well ahead of the orientee's first day in the department. The manager and preceptor must reschedule work to allow for the time it takes to effectively orient a new person. Don't expect the preceptor to handle a full work assignment *and* train an orientee. It can't be done well, and that attitude toward orientation leads to dissatisfaction and fast burnout for orientee and preceptor alike.

CONDUCTING THE ORIENTATION

The First Day

The department head should personally welcome the new employee. If a supervisor is directly responsible for the orientee, he or she guides the first day's progress, even if a preceptor is used. An orientation packet gives the new person material to refer back to later, and shows that the department is well-prepared and well-organized (see Exhibit 6–6 for suggested contents). At periodic intervals during the day, assign material to be read. Aside from reinforcing vital information, these reading times offer a break from the constant interchange with other people. It can be a terrible strain to be concerned about making a good impression for eight straight hours. Sitting off in an office or a quiet corner reading can be a welcome relief. Just don't make these sessions too long. The notorious "give 'em the policy book and get 'em out of the way for the rest of the day" approach to orientation should not be resurrected.

At some point during the day, the manager needs to sit down with the orientee and reaffirm the goals and objectives of orientation. Ask for feedback about the person's own feelings and expectations. Cften the most conscientious and hard-working employees doubt their competency as they see the department functioning at full productivity and co-workers performing with intimidating efficiency. The following quotation should be engraved in letters of fire on the consciousness of orientees, their supervisors, and their co-workers: "No matter how able, experienced, and concerned the new employee, he cannot perform at full productivity in a strange work situation until he becomes familiar with the physical layout, the people, the procedures, the regulations, the channels, and the equipment around him."[6]

Talented, promising orientees will be lost to the department and the organization unless their managers make it clear that new people are not expected to perform as well or as efficiently as experienced workers for quite some time. Reinforce and validate this statement by keeping work assignments small for a while, so that neither orientees nor the work group can compare output.

Teaching Job Activities

As job training begins, find out what the new employee already knows about the work. Then individualize instruction to prevent repetition of known material. It is vital to explain why the job is important and how it contributes to the overall hospital mission of quality patient care. Don't assume new employees know this—often they do not.

Exhibit 6–6 Department Orientation Packet Contents

Schedule of orientation

Memorandum announcing employment

Job description

List of pertinent JCAH regulations

Department goals and objectives

Orientation checklist

Personnel information

Probationary evaluation form

Department rules and regulations

Telephone directory

Pertinent sample forms

Whether job instruction is carried out by instructor, manager, or co-worker, the following guidelines apply:

1. Demonstrate the job one step at a time, explaining the reasons behind each step.
2. Limit instructions so that the employee is not overwhelmed. Don't give alternate ways of doing it at first. Concentrate on the one best way.
3. Have the orientee try each step, explaining the key points back to you. Be sure the rationale is understood, rather than the orientee just repeating by rote.
4. Indicate when performance is correct.
5. Correct errors immediately. Don't let a mistake become a habit.
6. Take nothing for granted. Although you can do the job in your sleep, the new employee is bound to have questions, even if none are asked. Many people are afraid of appearing dumb or slow to catch on, and will nod their head obligingly if you say "Do you understand?" or give a negative shake to the query "Any questions?" *You* ask the questions to check understanding. And let the orientee know that questions about the job indicate thoughtfulness and interest.

It is a good idea to encourage new people to bring their questions to the supervisor if no designated preceptor or instructor is used. Often other employees will give misleading or incomplete answers simply because they don't want to admit that they don't understand the question or know the answer. Taking questions to the supervisor results in correct information and reinforces the concept of the supervisor as resource and support person.

Another thing to encourage is active learning by new employees. Have them take notes during instruction and review them later. When a question arises that is covered in resource material such as the department policy book, help them look up the answer themselves. Introduce all new people to the hospital library, and demonstrate its use as a self-study resource. Anything you can do to communicate the idea that each person is responsible for personal development will yield the long-term benefits of well-informed, independent employees.

Completing Orientation

Limit early assignments, both to prevent the employee from being overwhelmed and to ensure success. These small assignments should be very gradually increased until the orientee is carrying a full load. The use of an orientation checklist prevents skipping important information as the training period progresses (see Exhibit 6–7 for an example). As the employee gains confidence and performs well with the full assignment, gradually decrease supervision. Don't simply turn the orientee loose—just follow less and less closely over a period of days and weeks, depending on job complexity and demonstrated ability.

This process cannot be rushed. For most jobs with any complexity, three to six months are probably needed for an employee to perform satisfactorily and fully understand the job. If insufficient time is devoted to developing orientees, poor performance and decreased satisfaction will result. Remember, training is never really finished—even experienced employees need observation and follow-up to ensure continued excellence.

Be careful not to give the new person too much independence. One researcher found that autonomy or working alone actually creates dissatisfaction among new employees.[7] Orientees need support, praise, and interaction as they learn the formal and informal rules of operation and their individual roles in the organization.

EVALUATING DEPARTMENT ORIENTATION

As the formal orientation period draws to a close, review each part of the program with the orientee—who should do most of the talking. Note any problems that occurred during induction so that they can be prevented next time. Ask for advice on helping other new employees. What could have been done better? What was on target?

Exhibit 6–7 Donor Center Orientation Checklist

Employee Name ____________________ Date of Hire ____________

	Date shown/ Instructor	*Performed/ Instructor*
I. Reception Area		
A. Personnel	______	______
B. Equipment	______	______
C. Forms	______	______
1. Community donor	______	______
2. Replacement donor	______	______
3. Autologous donor	______	______
4. Therapeutic phlebotomy	______	______
5. Supportive apheresis donor	______	______
6. Therapeutic apheresis donor	______	______
D. Files		
1. Whole blood donation	______	______
2. Therapeutic phlebotomy	______	______
3. Apheresis	______	______
4. Blood usage/replacement	______	______
II. Interview Area		
A. Personnel	______	______
B. Interview	______	______
C. Examination/equipment	______	______
D. Donor referral	______	______
E. Supplies		
III. Donor Room		
A. Personnel	______	______
B. Equipment	______	______
C. Whole blood donation	______	______
1. Recording/labeling	______	______
2. Preparation of scale	______	______
3. Arm preparation	______	______
4. Venipuncture	______	______
5. Termination of procedure	______	______
6. Donor recovery	______	______
7. Donor reaction		
D. Supplies	______	______
E. Canteen area	______	______

Source: Donor Center, Huntington Memorial Hospital, Pasadena, California. Reprinted with permission.

As part of this evaluation process, comment on the employee's progress and achievement of objectives. Hopefully, this feedback has been ongoing throughout the entire orientation, but this meeting provides an opportunity for a formal summation. Many institutions require a three-month evaluation of new employees, with a raise forthcoming if performance is satisfactory. Chapter 13 deals with the evaluation process in more detail.

CONCLUSION

Department orientation can be a strong force for excellence if done correctly. Unlike experienced employees, who are controlled by past performances, the new employee has a strong need to belong and is highly receptive to cues from the supervisor. In providing expectations about performance, the supervisor forms attitudes and inspires ambitions that the employee will carry throughout employment.[8] Umiker summarizes the whole process: "At the end of orientation, the orientee should be able to say it is the best she has ever participated in—or we have failed."[9]

Chapter 7 examines the need for bilingual orientation programs. If large numbers of non-English-speaking people are applying for jobs at your hospital, you had better be prepared to orient them successfully. The ins and outs of that process can be tricky—but the rewards are worth it.

NOTES

1. "Welcome Aboard!" *Dynamic Supervision in the Hospital* (Number 378), (Waterford, Conn.: Bureau of Business Practice, November 25, 1979), 3.

2. Gordon F. Shea, "Supervising New Employees," *Training and Development Journal* 36, no. 1 (January 1982): 50.

3. Dee Ann Gillies, *Nursing Management: A Systems Approach* (Philadelphia: W.B. Saunders Co., 1982), 205.

4. Robert A. Jones, "Good Starts for New Employees," *Supervisory Management* 27, no. 6 (June 1982): 9.

5. Loren B. Belker, *The First-Time Manager* (New York: AMACOM, 1978), 66.

6. Julius Yourman, "Orientation of New Employees," in *Improving the Effectiveness of Hospital Management*, ed. Addison C. Bennett (New York: Metromedia Analearn, 1972), 261.

7. "Welcome Aboard!" 9.

8. Charles J. Teplitz, "How the Right Example Can Help the New Recruit Make the Team," *Supervisory Management* 25, no. 5 (May 1980): 33.

9. William O. Umiker, "Do You Orient or Disorient Your New Employees?" *MLO* 12, no. 8 (August 1980): 132.

Chapter 7

Bilingual Orientation Programs

CULTURAL DIVERSITY IN THE UNITED STATES

Cultural diversity has been defined by Leininger as "the overt and covert differences among people of different population groups with respect to their values, beliefs, language, physical characteristics, and general patterns of behavior."[1] The United States has been fortunate to have many different ethnic groups settle in its cities and countryside, bringing new ideas and new ways of living to enrich its society. Indeed, unless of Native American origin, all inhabitants are members of those groups who came from afar to find a new life in a strange land.

This process of emigrating to seek the promise represented by the United States is still going on, bringing many people eager to work and raise families. Many may be unable to speak English or have only a limited English vocabulary. It is absurd for non-English-speaking persons to sit through a hospitalwide orientation session conducted in a language they can neither speak nor understand. What approach should be taken by hospitals to address the needs of these orientees?

When discussion about presenting orientation information in another language begins, someone is sure to raise objections: "It will cost too much," "None of the instructors speak that language," or the old reliable "Let 'em learn English!" Such objections are not only wrong, they are avoiding the issue. An organization is bound, legally and morally, to provide equal employment opportunities for all people. This includes orientation to the institution's policies and procedures. Offering orientation only to the employees who speak English is discriminatory. It is also bad business. The initial cost of setting up a bilingual program will be quickly recovered by reduced error and waste.

Non-English-speaking people offer a heritage of caring harmonious with the mission of a hospital. Effective orientation enables these employees to mesh with the organization and its goals, making them more productive and enhancing patient care. As we discuss bilingual orientation in more detail, we will focus on one ethnic group in order to use specific examples. If you are involved with a different group, investigate its cultural beliefs and values and apply them as you make your preparations for orientation.

SPANISH-SPEAKING EMPLOYEES

Spanish-speaking persons in the United States number 14.6 million, according to the 1980 census, and experts feel that they may be the largest minority group in this country by the end of the 1980s.[2] Since several terms refer to people of Spanish origin, in this book the following definitions will be used: *Mexican-American* refers to Mexican-born workers in the United States; *Chicano* refers to the first or second generation born in this country; *Hispanic* refers to anyone whose native language is Spanish (Mexicans, Cubans, Puerto Ricans, and South and Central Americans).

As an organization prepares to assimilate non-English-speaking workers into the system, certain questions arise:

1. Should bilingual classes be provided?
2. If so, who should provide them?
3. Could these orientees receive the information through handouts written in Spanish?

It cannot be stressed too strongly that orientation classes should be given in Spanish unless the number of orientees is very small. If only a few Hispanics are hired, orientation could be provided on a one-to-one basis. But if that proves impractical, bilingual classes are essential.

If no instructor speaks Spanish, a personnel representative or manager may have to teach the classes. Work with the responsible person to develop a program as effective and information filled as regular new employee orientation. Resist the complaint that this is duplication and "if they're going to work here they should learn English." Professor Pastora San Juan of the University of Chicago suggests that, because Mexico lies just across the United States border and Mexican-Americans tend to migrate back and forth in three- to seven-year cycles, the cultural conflict is even stronger than for other immigrants.[3] Many Mexican-Americans who would like to speak English find it difficult because economic conditions in their home country required them to work, thus restricting educational opportunities. One study found that almost 27 percent of Mexican-origin persons 25 or older had completed less than five years of school (the corresponding rate for the total United States population was 4.6 percent).[4]

The answer to the third question seems self-evident: no orientation should be given entirely by handout. Certainly some handouts should be used, but to offer a second-rate orientation simply because the orientees affected do not speak English is clearly a policy based on ethnocentrism (the belief that one's own beliefs, values, and lifeways are superior to or more desirable than the life styles of others[5]).

Before planning a bilingual orientation, investigate the components of the other culture so you can incorporate some of the values and beliefs of the participants into the classes. For instance, several aspects of Hispanic culture have a major impact on employment and orientation:

1. In the dominant culture of the United States, being responsible is equated with being on time for appointments. The Hispanic may not be so locked in to the clock, since the concept of responsibility is based on other values (particularly meeting family needs).[6]
2. Persons with Anglo backgrounds are taught to value frank, direct expression of thoughts and feelings. The traditional Latin approach is based on tact and respect for the other's feelings, which often requires much circumlocution to always provide a way to preserve dignity.[7]
3. Anglo-Americans often express their affection for others by kidding them. A reunion of old friends, for example, may start off with a round of good-natured insults. Hispanics may find kidding offensive and see it as rude and deprecating. When offering criticism of any kind to someone of Latin descent, care must be taken to phrase the statement with respect to dignity and saving face. Murillo states, "There seems to be a high degree of vulnerability to almost any kind of criticism on the part of Latins everywhere."[8]

Implications for Orientation

How should bilingual orientation be planned to take into consideration cultural factors affecting adjustment to the hospital? Very little has been done to research this problem in work settings. One study of Spanish-speaking students in a nursing program has implications for hospital orientation. With respect to difficulties adjusting to the program, 58 percent indicated that language caused the most problems; 50 percent said there was too much content to be absorbed in a short period of time; and 33 percent said the program was extremely competitive and not flexible as to student needs. Of the factors that would help adjustment, the top two listed were a good orientation program and a mutual understanding of cultural background.[9]

Providing bilingual orientation should help with the language problems, and content overload is a constant obstacle to guard against. But what about competitiveness and inflexibility? At first glance they might be dismissed as potential trouble spots. But take another look—from what viewpoint is competitiveness and flexibility being judged? The North American culture encourages competitiveness and individuality, while some other cultures emphasize noncompetitiveness and group learning. A quick review of Chapter 4 will demonstrate that many teaching strategies are based on the dominant features of learning in the United States. Wong and Wong caution that "faculty who are firm believers in the independent learning style must be cautious of using this technique with the ethnic minority students."[10]

Your orientation presentation should link the culture to the information being presented. Hemans makes the following suggestions:

1. Get the basic need-to-know information about their jobs right up front.
2. Make your presentations visual whenever possible.
3. Go easy on the reading—and when handouts are used, be sure the illustrations aren't all Anglo people.
4. Use role play and simulations as you would in any training situation, save that you want to be unusually concrete in the message.
5. If you pose examples which relate to their culture, the participants will remember those examples a long time.[11]

Work with the person who will be making the presentation in the other language, whether employee representative, counselor, or manager. Crucial items such as hospital performance expectations, how payroll deductions are made for taxes, social security, insurance, and other items, and a detailed explanation of benefits must be addressed. One Hispanic worker commented "We need better explanations in simple terms. Like they should tell us how to use the insurance and how to use the benefits. We don't know this at all so it is just like we don't have insurance."[12]

Other helpful items to be explained include how to find public transportation and car pools, what safety and work rules must be followed, and how to use the hospital grievance procedures. Some mechanism must be provided to clue the orientees in to what's expected as far as reporting to work on time, taking breaks and lunch, and other rules and mores of the work group. In the work area, bulletin board notices, cartoons, and signs in clear English and Spanish may be effective.

Communicating

As we have noted, many Mexican-Americans do not read Spanish well.[13] Therefore, extensive use of written material to pass on important information is not recommended. Anything vital should be reinforced verbally, not just given in writing.

One important thing to keep in mind when preparing bilingual handouts or employee manuals is that mistranslations can occur. A study on Hispanic responses to questionnaires found that when the questionnaire was written in English and then translated into Spanish, incorrect idiom was used in several instances. Follow-up interviews with some respondents revealed that these translation problems generally only caused amusement, but on at least one occasion a potentially serious misunderstanding resulted.[14] These data indicate that translations must be made as closely equivalent to the original source as possible. The recommended way to achieve this is back-translation—after the first translation is completed, the Spanish version should be translated back into English by someone other than the original translator. This translation-back-translation process should be repeated until an English translation is made that closely matches the original.

Another method of conveying important information to non-English-speaking employees is through the use of audiocassettes. In one hospital, audiocassettes in different languages have been successfully used to inform patients about hospital activities, such as preoperative routines, postoperative care, and preparation for diagnostic tests.[15] This concept could be expanded to include a library of audiocassettes for employees explaining key benefits, policies, and procedures in Spanish or other languages. If a non-English-speaking employee had a question, quick reference to the appropriate tape might provide the answer. Although no substitute for a Spanish-speaking employee representative in the personnel department, such a tape collection could certainly provide support on the evening and night shifts and on weekends and holidays.

Help for Supervisors

If the hospital has supervisors working with employees of other cultures, some information about the values and beliefs of the workers is helpful. This information could be presented in a workshop or in a series of meetings with the appropriate supervisors. Using the workshop format would enable participants to try role playing and other techniques designed to put them in the worker's shoes for a while.

As examples of what might be covered, consider the following information about Mexican-American employees:

1. These workers try hard to be productive, considering it high praise to be called "muy trabajador"—hard worker.
2. Nearly all Mexican workers prefer a supervisor who explains everything down to the last detail; they want explicit directions and very structured tasks.
3. Often these employees regard the supervisor as a father-figure or teacher, and these authority figures should demonstrate good manners and serious-

ness. Joking, kidding, or yelling at workers when something goes wrong are all likely to be resented.

4. When correction is necessary, Mexican workers wish to be corrected plainly and patiently, as a father or teacher would do.[16]

Of course, these examples all relate to good management practices with any employee, regardless of cultural background. Providing a cultural rationale for such actions may help the supervisors relate to their necessity and the payoffs linked to such behavior. Raising people's consciousness about cultural factors impacting on productivity may start them thinking about interpersonal relations in supervision of all employees.

Programs for Ethnic Workers

In most organizations in the United States, promotion is dependent on the ability to speak English. To provide opportunities for minority employees, the hospital should investigate possibilities for teaching courses in English as a Second Language (ESL). Community agencies are often ready to conduct these programs on company or organization premises. Courses are readily available in New York, Detroit, Chicago, Los Angeles, Cleveland, and Newark. The Hartford Hospital in Connecticut instituted a program with trained employees who volunteered to teach ESL to Hispanic co-workers; to date this has proven very successful.[17]

The advantages of conducting onsite programs include convenience for the learners and an adult approach to learning. Attendance at ''school'' can be embarrassing for adults. The relaxed, practical approach to learning English will not only be appreciated by participants, it will encourage attendance and learning. And while you are arranging English as a Second Language course for your non-English-speaking employees, why not set up Spanish or other language courses for the English-speaking staff? Bilingualism can facilitate patient and family relations as well as staff communication.

CONCLUSION

Providing bilingual orientation for non-English-speaking employees will benefit the organization as much as the workers. The planner should adapt teaching techniques to the cultural values and beliefs of the target group, and should ensure that any written material is accurate both grammatically and factually.

If information on employee expectations and values is communicated to the responsible supervisors, on-the-job relations and productivity will both improve. The hospital can encourage development of minority workers by providing English as a Second Language classes at the work site.

NOTES

1. Madeleine Leininger, ''Cultural Diversity of Health and Nursing Care,'' *Nursing Clinics of North America* 12, no. 1 (March 1977): 9.

2. Mariah E. deForest, ''Mexican Workers North of the Border,'' *Harvard Business Review* 59, no. 3 (May-June 1981): 150.

3. Ibid., 152.

4. Ibid.

5. Leininger, ''Cultural Diversity,'' 11.

6. Nathan Murillo, ''The Mexican-American Family,'' in *Hispanic Culture and Health Care: Fact, Fiction, and Folklore,* ed. Ricardo Arguijo Martinez (St. Louis: C.V. Mosby Co., 1978): 8.

7. Ibid.

8. Ibid., 9.

9. Huda Abu-Saad, Jeanie Kayser-Jones, and Yolanda Gutierrez, ''Latin American Nursing Students in the United States,'' *Journal of Nursing Education* 21, no. 7 (September 1982): 19.

10. Shirley Wong and Julia Wong, ''Problems in Teaching Ethnic Minority Nursing Students,'' *Journal of Advanced Nursing* 7, (1982): 258.

11. H. Hemans, ''The Minority Volunteers,'' *Health Care Education* 9 (April-May 1980): 27.

12. deForest, ''Mexican Workers,'' 152.

13. Ibid., 153.

14. Emil Berkanovic, ''The Effect of Inadequate Language Translation on Hispanics' Responses to Health Surveys,'' *American Journal of Public Health* 70, no. 12 (December 1980): 1276.

15. Jay Melrose, ''Audiocassettes Help Hospitals Break Language Barriers to Care,'' *Hospitals, J.A.H.A.* 51 (November 1, 1977): 93.

16. deForest, ''Mexican Workers,'' 152.

17. Ibid., 156.

Part III

Nursing Orientation

Chapter 8

Nursing Orientation in the Classroom

Nursing orientation is usually much longer than orientation of allied personnel. Hospitals have provided formal programs for nurses for a number of years—only lately have other employees also received classes. Because of this history, nursing orientation is traditionally more elaborate.

JCAH lists its guidelines for general nursing orientation as follows:

> New nursing department/service personnel shall receive an orientation of sufficient duration and content to prepare them for their specific duties and responsibilities in the hospital. The orientation shall be based on the educational needs identified by assessment of the individual's ability, knowledge, and skills. Any necessary instruction shall be provided nursing service personnel before they administer direct patient care.[1]

COORDINATING THE PROGRAM

To carry out this responsibility, one person from the education department should be designated as the coordinator for nursing orientation. Fredericks found that when systems for providing orientation are inadequate there are a number of reasons: (1) insufficient time, (2) inadequate communication between those hiring and those responsible for orienting and supervising new employees, (3) lack of follow-up, and (4) insufficient information about roles and expectations.[2] An orientation coordinator can set up information channels to transmit preemployment information to educators and supervisors and to share plans for orienting new nurses.

The head nurse is ultimately responsible for planning and implementing orientation. But every organization has certain core knowledge that is needed by employees before they can function within their designated positions.[3] Dissemination of this critical information is the duty of the centralized education department, specifically, of the designated orientation coordinator.

SCHEDULING

In order to present the core information in an organized way, nursing orientation should be scheduled to coincide with hospitalwide orientation. This prevents repetition of information and reinforces the important points covered in new employee orientation. Notice that scheduling nursing orientation as an immediate follow-up to the hospitalwide program implies a biweekly or twice a month interval between groups. This is crucial: *schedule* orientation to begin on specific dates. Orienting nurses as they are hired not only carries a strong flavor of desperation ("Just work for us; we'll orient you anytime!"), it also ensures a disorganized presentation of material, confused or nonexistent guest speakers, and an orientation instructor headed for burnout.

The easiest way to achieve perfect scheduling is for all managers, working in cooperation with the personnel department, to hire new people to begin on predetermined start dates. After the hiring decision is made, the head nurse consults a calendar for the next scheduled orientation and instructs the new employee to begin work on that date. Personnel representatives then complete the paperwork and give the orientee a letter of welcome from the orientation coordinator (see Exhibit 8–1) and a list of the content covered in the program. At the designated time on the start date, the orientee reports to the classroom listed in the letter and orientation begins.

If you can persuade the managers that such organized scheduling leads to a better prepared, less anxious employee, coordinating orientation will be easy and pleasant. If not, at least hold firm on set start dates for orientation. Then when a new nurse is hired and the head nurse insists on an immediate start, the orientee can work on the unit with a partner (never unsupervised) until going into the next scheduled orientation. The potential for error and confusion is great in this approach, but you may have little choice.

Whichever approach is used, the coordinator should receive the names of new people as soon as possible. In most hospitals these names are provided by Personnel. Ask that you be given the list of orientees as far in advance as possible, remembering that additions may be made later. The minimum information needed about each orientee is

1. Name
2. Start date
3. Position classification (RN, NA, US, etc.)

Exhibit 8–1 Letter to Nursing Orientees

Dear Orientee:

Welcome to Hometown Community Hospital! When you begin work on ________________, please report to Room ______________ promptly at 8:00 A.M. A copy of the orientation schedule is included for your information. Note that no uniforms are required until Friday.

During the first week you will take a pharmacology test designed to evaluate your ability to calculate dosages and IV drip rates, as well as your knowledge of common drug actions. This test must be passed before you can administer medications. If not passed the first time it must be retaken and passed by the end of the second week of orientation.

Please bring a pen or pencil with you to all orientation classes. Orientation is designed to provide the information you need to assume your new role in this hospital, so come prepared to learn and enjoy. Our responsibility is to offer all the information and help that we can; your responsibility is to absorb the information and apply it to your practice.

If you have any questions about orientation classes or their scheduling, please call the Education Department at ________________. We're looking forward to seeing you!

Sincerely,

Orientation Coordinator

4. Unit
5. Shift
6. Full time/part time

It is also helpful to know something about the background and experience of each orientee, but this can be discovered once orientation has begun.

With the information provided by Personnel, the coordinator can then prepare the schedules. The easiest way to do this is to use standard schedules which are then personalized for each orientee by typing in name, unit, and pertinent dates (see Exhibit 8–2). Make a copy for the orientee, the manager, the unit preceptor, the orientation instructor, and the staffing office. This simple schedule is the single most powerful communication tool you have. Use it to prevent misunderstandings about what the orientee will be doing when.

In the system we are using as an example, nursing orientation lasts three weeks for a nurse with previous work experience. There is no magic number of hours, days, or weeks required to produce a confident, well-oriented practitioner. Later in the chapter competency-based and modular programs will be discussed, neither of which have set times for completion. The length and schedule should depend on the hospital's requirements and the nurse's needs.

Exhibit 8–2 Nursing Orientation Schedule

RN/LVN Orientation Schedule

Orientee __________ **Head Nurse** __________
Unit __________ **Orientation Instructor** __________

Monday	Tuesday	Wednesday	Thursday	Friday
8:00–4:30 EDUC. DEPT. 8:00–2:30 New Employee Orientation 2:30–4:30 Unit (Observation)	8:00–4:30 EDUC. DEPT. Nursing Orientation Classes	8:00–4:30 EDUC. DEPT. Basic Cardiac Support	8:00–4:30 EDUC. DEPT. 8:00–11:00 New Employee Orientation 11:00–11:45 Lunch 11:45–4:30 Nursing Orientation	7:00–3:30 UNIT Patient Care (Buddy System) (UNIFORMS)
8:00–4:30 EDUC. DEPT. Nursing Orientation Classes	8:00–4:30 EDUC. DEPT. Nursing Orientation Classes	7:00–3:30 UNIT Work with U.S. and Charge Nurse on CRT and Desk	7:00–3:30 UNIT Total Patient Care (2–3 patients)	7:00–3:30 UNIT Total Patient Care (3–4 patients)
7:00–3:30 UNIT Work Buddy System with Team Leader	7:00–3:30 UNIT Work as Team Leader for ½ Team	7:00–3:30 UNIT Full Team Leading	7:00–3:30 UNIT Full Team Leading	7:00–3:30 UNIT Full Team Leading (Go to unit schedule)

Source: Education Department, Huntington Memorial Hospital, Pasadena, California. Reprinted with permission.

PLANNING CONTENT

The content of nursing orientation should be selected according to the results of the needs assessment conducted as discussed in Chapter 2. Once you know what information is needed, sequencing the content is the next step. Data required by all nurses should be presented in centralized orientation classes; those facts specific to particular areas should be covered at the unit level. For example, orientees working in critical care would learn how to record information on the basic chart during centralized classes. They would learn how to use critical care flowsheets and forms after they reach the unit.

Setting priorities for presenting content should be based on overall orientation objectives. Refer to Exhibit 3–1 in Chapter 3 for an example of overall program objectives—behaviors expected from participants when orientation is completed. Cantor states that "those activities most crucial to the patient's welfare should come earliest in the training sequence."[4]

Another way of sequencing information includes consideration of progressive development and continuity of content. Blocks of facts should build upon one another in a logical, reinforcing manner. Segall lists some guidelines for this process:

1. Are course segments prerequisite to others introduced prior to those others?
2. Are there any units or activities that might facilitate the total learning experience by occurring early?
3. Are there segments within different units which may be confusing if taught separately, and should be taught at the same time?
4. Might students be motivated by a demonstration of certain skills at a high level of simulation before they practice those skills at a lower level of simulation?[5]

Most of these guidelines are self-explanatory, but an example illustrating the last one might prove helpful. When teaching CPR, instructors demonstrate perfect technique before bringing the students into groups to practice the skills. Observing CPR done properly enables students to model their practice, gives a goal to work toward, and validates instructor expertise.

Learning activities should also be sequenced to maintain orientee interest and motivation. When selecting teaching strategies, try to achieve a mix of information delivery and active participation. Exhibit 8–3 lists the content sequence and timing for some nursing orientation classes. Choosing the first Tuesday as an example, notice that the day opens with a presentation of nursing department organization by the director of nursing. This involves discussion and sharing of background and experience—an instant attention getter that makes it an ideal way

Exhibit 8–3 Sample Sequence of Nursing Orientation

Revised Orientation Content

First Week

Monday 8:00 A.M. to 4:00 P.M.

8:00 – 12:00	New employee orientation
12:00 – 1:00	Lunch with unit staff
1:00 – 2:30	Introduction to C.A.R.E.S.
2:30 – 3:00	Review of schedules and packets
3:00 – 3:45	Tour of first floor
3:45 – 4:30	Pharmacology test

Tuesday 8:00 A.M. to 4:30 P.M.

8:00 – 9:00	Organization of the nursing department
9:00 – 10:00	Infection control
10:00 – 10:15	Break
10:15 – 11:30	Patient evacuation
11:30 – 12:15	Lunch
12:15 – 1:00	Disaster game
1:00 – 2:00	Charting (forms and introduction to systematic assessment)
2:00 – 2:15	Break
2:15 – 3:15	Nursing care plans
3:15 – 3:45	Charting practice (untoward incidents)
3:45 – 4:30	Tour of ground and basement

Wednesday 8:00 A.M. to 4:30 P.M.

8:00 – 4:30	Basic cardiac life support

Thursday 8:00 A.M. to 4:30 P.M.

8:00 – 11:00	New employee orientation
11:00 – 11:45	Patient mobility
11:45 – 12:30	Lunch
12:30 – 1:30	Legal implications
1:30 – 2:45	Medication administration and charting
2:45 – 3:00	Break
3:00 – 3:45	Charting practice (admissions)
3:45 – 4:30	Tour of 2, 3, and 4.

Second Week

Monday 8:00 A.M. to 4:30 P.M.

8:00 – 11:15	CRT class in C.A.R.E.S.
11:15 – 12:00	Lunch
12:00 – 1:15	Charting review (discharges and general critiques)
1:15 – 2:00	Respiratory therapy
2:00 – 2:15	Break
2:15 – 3:00	Dietary
3:00 – 3:30	Radiology
3:30 – 4:30	Manual self-study

Exhibit 8–3 continued

Tuesday 8:00 A.M. to 4:30 P.M.	
8:00 – 11:15	CRT class in C.A.R.E.S.
11:15 – 12:00	Lunch
12:00 – 1:00	Charting practice (general assessment and documentation)
1:00 – 1:30	Patient services
1:30 – 1:45	Break
1:45 – 2:15	Quality Assurance
2:15 – 3:30	IV maintenance and charting
3:30 – 4:30	Manual self-study

to open the day. Infection control is lecture/demonstration. Patient evacuation requires return demonstration of patient carries, so participants are up and moving. After lunch people often feel sleepy, so a competitive game is placed in that time slot. A lecture-discussion of charting forms and systematic patient assessment is followed by a badly needed break. Rather than listen to a lecture about care plans, the class divides into small groups and actually develops care plans for some simulated patients, drawing on the orientees' experience and previous knowledge of this subject. Then charting practice is provided when their hypothetical patients become involved in some startling situations. The day ends with a tour of part of the facility in order to provide a low-pressure finale.

Further examination of this schedule reveals that the nurses are not sent to the units until they have some background in activities crucial to patient welfare: infection control, evacuation, fire safety, charting, care plans, CPR, and medication administration. Material on intravenous fluids, lines, and maintenance is presented later, but orientees do not handle IVs until they have had that class. The reinforcement and logical sequencing can be seen in the progressively more difficult charting practice and reviews, each of which builds on previous content.

In this example, full-day orientation classes are given. It can be argued that learning would take place more readily if classes lasted only four hours, with the remaining four hours spent on the unit (or reversing this, spending the first four hours giving care and going to class in the afternoon). This, too, can be done, but several factors must be kept in mind. First, unless the orientees are only helping with another nurse's assignment, someone has to cover their patients when they're gone. This tends to make both staff and manager regard orientees as a burden rather than a help. Second, most orientees find it difficult to leave their patients to go to class, which creates late arrivals or even absences. If the class is given in the morning, coming on to the unit in the afternoon means "observing," since there is little else they can do at that time of day—they certainly can't take a patient assignment. And most important, orientees tend to resent split scheduling, complaining that it drags out the process interminably, delays needed information, fragments their socialization with unit personnel, and makes them feel like students again.

CONDUCTING ORIENTATION CLASSES

Who teaches orientation classes? For the sake of consistency of information, the orientation coordinator is the best person to conduct all nursing orientation sessions. But many people find it hard to teach the same content over and over again, so in most hospitals these classes are shared by all nursing instructors. The burden of organizing this effort must be borne by the coordinator, however. Schedules must be made out and distributed, rooms and refreshments arranged, guest speakers confirmed, packets put together. And most important, all instructors must be constantly updated as to changes in policy, new equipment and procedures, and any other information impacting on the orientation process.

When meeting orientees for the first time, which generally happens at the end of new employee orientation, instructors must work to establish a professional, helping climate. Remember that these are adult learners, so a schoolroom atmosphere should be avoided. The first thing orientees want to know is what will be happening to them, so go over the schedules and answer questions about orientation as a whole. Pass out packets and review the contents, which generally include:

1. Job description
2. List of key people in the nursing division
3. Skills inventory
4. If used, a survey of learning needs
5. Handouts pertinent to nursing orientation. Everything that will be used during the classes can be given out in the beginning, in handbook form, or individual class handouts can be given out at the time of use. A large bound handbook is generally more convenient for the instructor and learner (just be sure to number the pages for quick reference), since it helps prevent the loss of important material.

Give clear instructions on how to find meeting places and whether uniforms are required for classes. A review of parking areas is usually appreciated at this point, and be sure to tell the orientees that refreshments will be provided at the beginning of class, so they won't buy their own coffee and bring it to the classroom.

Orientation Testing

In that first meeting you should discuss the hospital's policy about any testing to be done, such as the pharmacology test. This should have been explained during

Exhibit 8–4 Sample Orientation Examination Policy

> During the three-week orientation period all nurses are required to take and pass the hospital pharmacology examination before being allowed to administer medications. Any nurse who does not achieve a passing score (80%) must repeat the examination. If the second test is also failed, the nurse must take the one-week pharmacology course offered by the education department. After taking the course, the nurse will be required to retake the examination. If the test is again failed, employment will be terminated. This entire process must be completed before the end of the probationary period.

the hiring interview, but check for understanding and answer questions. Best of all, provide each orientee with a copy of the written policy, straight from the Policy Manual. This policy should be set by nursing administration and must apply equally to all newly hired nurses. Exhibit 8–4 is an example of such a policy. Notice that the responsibility for learning the needed knowledge is placed on the orientee. The instructor's role is to guide orientees to resources for self-study and to answer questions. In a hospital where failirg to pass the pharmacology test means automatic enrollment in a pharmacology course, the instructor might be responsible for scheduling the person in the next course. In either case, communicating test results to the head nurse is essential, since the hospital's responsibility for each employee's safe practice demands that no nurse be allowed to administer drugs without some minimum skill level being ascertained.

When should the test be given? Some people feel it should be completed on the very first day, with little or no warning. Others believe that this is inappropriate, since orientees are usually exhausted at that point. The test should be designed to measure acceptable knowledge of dosage calculation and drug data (determined by validating the test with current staff, as discussed in Chapter 2). Since you are trying to determine the level of knowledge that nurses enter the institution with, will results be skewed by "cramming" the night before the test? That is the fear expressed by people who feel it should be given on the first day. Opponents feel that a properly designed test will measure competency to calculate dosages and knowledge of drug actions and interactions regardless of any studying done by the testee. This issue should be decided by the people involved before instituting a policy.

Class Sessions

In setting up the class, maintain an adult learner-centered atmosphere. In some settings, this can be difficult. If desk chairs are available, arrange them in a semicircle rather than classroom-style. If you have tables and chairs, try a U-shape setup. It seems almost unnecessary to stress the importance of having coffee, tea, and decaffeinated coffee available; such refreshments are vital. Don't wait until the break—the beverages should be available first thing. If the hospital provides doughnuts or rolls, a clear message of concern is conveyed. If not, see if you can arrange for some hot chocolate packets—these are usually appreciated by everyone.

Relevance of information is maintained by stressing its relationship to patient care. If you cannot demonstrate how the content will contribute to improving care, leave it out. One effective way to highlight importance is through orientee participation. What makes this essential information? How have the learners used it in the past? How will they use it on the unit? Have the orientees identify and explain content relevance based on their own experience. Whatever is being covered will impact much more strongly when the learners relate it to personal practice. In effect, the more the orientees teach each other the content, the better it will be retained.

As classes progress, the schedule becomes more and more important. It should be designed so that each topic can be covered in the time allowed. Once the instructor has to take "just a few minutes" to finish material from the day before, the whole structure of orientation will come tumbling down. How can you allow enough time for each subject? Write careful objectives for each individual segment. In the initial assessment you determined what information was needed by orientees; the overall orientation objectives determined the end behaviors necessary for each learner. With the individual class objectives you now limit content to that which is necessary to achieve the objectives. This process is vital when time is a factor, as it always is in orientation. When there isn't enough time to properly cover all topics, it is tempting to try to teach all content in the time allowed. As Broadwell points out, such an approach invalidates the objectives.[6] If less time is available than is needed to teach all the material, revise the objectives, eliminating some of the lower priority content.

Exhibit 8–5 is an example of individual class objectives. Although all the content is important, objectives 1, 2, 3, 4, and 9 have the highest priority, since they directly affect practice. If a lecture format was used, those might be the only ones covered in the one hour allotted for this class. However, converting the information into a pretest, which is then reviewed and discussed, not only allows every point to be covered, it also eliminates repetition of material that the participants already know. Discussion stems from questions and comments made as the correct answers are reviewed; if everyone is familiar with the point being covered, no time need be spent on it.

Using participants to teach content reinforces their knowledge of patient care and validates individual expertise. One way to do this is in a class that is essentially review, but where it is vital that all nurses be able to perform correctly. Exhibit 8–6 shows a set of objectives for a class on patient mobility. Each participant receives a

Exhibit 8–5 Individual Class Objectives

Legal Implications

Objectives

After participating in this session, the orientee will be able to:

1. Correctly and completely fill out a Notification Form.
2. Correctly and completely fill out a Report of Medication Error Form.
3. Explain what should be charted in the Nurses Notes when an incident occurs.
4. List the steps to be followed if an employee is injured while at work.
5. State the reasons for carrying malpractice insurance.
6. Define the following and explain the implications each has for nursing.

    a. Assault
    b. Battery
    c. False imprisonment
    d. Confidentiality
    e. Negligence/Malpractice
    f. Standard of care

7. Discuss legal rationales for recording patient information.
8. Explain the concept of "Respondeat Superior" and how it affects nurses.
9. List the steps to follow when questioning a physician's order.

Source: Education Department, Huntington Memorial Hospital, Pasadena, California. Reprinted with permission.

Exhibit 8–6 Patient Mobility Objectives

By the end of the session, the participant will be able to:

1. Transfer a patient from bed to wheelchair and back again using safe body mechanics to avoid injury.
2. Turn the patient in bed in a way that provides patient comfort and safety and protects the nurse.
3. Move a patient up in bed without causing shearing pressure.
4. Move a patient who has slid down in a chair to an upright position without back strain.
5. Demonstrate proper positioning for an immobilized patient in the following positions:
    a. Side-lying
    b. Prone
6. Demonstrate proper use of the following devices:
    a. Foot splint
    b. Hand roll
    c. Positioning devices such as trochanter rolls and foam blocks
7. Demonstrate complete range-of-motion exercises for an immobilized patient.
8. Ambulate a patient to provide maximum patient safety.

copy. The group then divides into teams of two or three and each team is assigned to demonstrate one or more objectives, depending on the number of teams. Resource material on patient mobility and the hospital procedure manual are available for reference. After the teams have had a chance to practice their demonstrations, the group gets back together and each objective is presented. Discussion centers on the rationale for each technique, and anyone unfamiliar with a certain method can practice with feedback from the team responsible. This teaching technique results in high levels of learner interest and motivation, as well as providing a test of knowledge and practice.

Tours

A different approach to learning necessary content relates to the obligatory tours of the hospital. Generally, the larger the hospital, the less orientees will remember of any tour. If an actual tour is necessary, break these excursions into a series of minitours, each covering a small part of the physical plant. Everything pointed out during tours should relate to the orientees' daily practice. Do the nurses really need to know where the doctor's lounge is during the first week? If it's not necessary to what they'll be doing, don't include it.

Some hospitals are trying a different approach to orienting new employees to the layout of the institution. Feeling that the only way to become familiar with a hospital is to explore it on one's own, these organizations have designed scavenger hunts that are both learning and socializing experiences. Exhibit 8–7 is an example of one such device. Notice that the number of other departments that must be located is limited to areas the nurse might need to find in the first days of the new job. Other places, such as Purchasing, Carpenter Shop, or Telecommunications can wait until the new employee is more familiar with the total institution. On the individual unit the things to be found are those needed to deliver safe patient care—not a complete list, but a good beginning. Time for the hunt should be provided during the orientation class; this kind of activity makes a good after-lunch session. Some hospitals use a check-in system for the scavenger hunt, with the orientees picking up cards, chips, or signatures from people in each area they tour.

Guest Speakers

How many guest speakers do you use in nursing orientation? All too often the program is loaded with presenters from other departments because "nurses need to know how that department works" or because those people have *always* spoken in nursing orientation. Take time to scrutinize this involvement. Certainly, nurses need to know how other departments contribute to patient care and interface with

Exhibit 8–7 Scavenger Hunt

This is your opportunity to locate items and areas that you will utilize in your work. Please make good use of the allotted time. Try to locate items on your own, but if you can't, ask for assistance.

Ground floor
- Emergency Department
- Pathology and Morgue
- Physical Therapy
- Central Sterile Supply

First floor
- Library
- Nursing Office
- Staffing Office
- In-patient Pharmacy
- Surgery waiting lounge
- Radiology
- Cashier

Second floor
- CCU
- ICU
- Recovery Room

Third floor
- Clinical laboratories

Your nursing station
- Fire exits
- Fire alarms
- Fire extinguishers
- Crash cart
- Portable oxygen
- Syringes
- Allergy sticker
- Time sheet
- Medication carts
- Policy/Procedure manuals
- IV solutions
- Scale
- Wheelchairs
- Chart forms
- Sitz bath
- Blankets
- Narcotic record book
- Showers
- Toilet paper
- Satellite pharmacy
- Chux

Source: Education Department, Huntington Memorial Hospital, Pasadena, California. Reprinted by permission.

nursing. For instance, every nurse needs to know when and how to communicate with the dietary department, or how to order treatments from respiratory services, or how to call in a social worker to help patients and their families. But how much do nurses need to learn during orientation? Often guest speakers from other departments add so much extraneous material to their talks that the essentials are obscured and ultimately lost. Cantor states that:

> It is important to realize that members of other departments will look at the nurse's educational needs in terms of their own jobs, the content associated with their own specialties, and the values they hold in relation to their positions. The extent to which their areas of knowledge are appropriate for nurses can be determined only by nurses.[7]

The needs assessment you performed at the start should help with this determination. Once the necessary information has been selected, decide who should present it. Often it can be presented in an appropriate and timely manner by the orientation instructor. If a guest speaker is used in order to foster good relations between departments or because the orientees need to know the speaker, very specific objectives should be given to the guest. These objectives should delineate exactly what needs to be covered. A time limit set by the orientation instructor should be explained to the speaker. You then must be ready to step in and enforce this limit if the speaker goes over it. If this happens a few times, guests quickly realize the seriousness of time constraints and streamline their presentations.

As the person responsible for the learning and beginning performance of the orientees, the instructor must not hesitate to replace a speaker if necessary. Presenters who are nervous or boring can often be helped, but one who exhibits contempt for the audience should be promptly eliminated. Once a guest speaker actually stated that nurses should not "interfere" in patient care by suctioning or adjusting the ties for a patient with a tracheotomy, as only respiratory therapists were capable of doing these procedures correctly. The orientation instructor promptly intervened by pointing out that hospital policy permitted nurses to perform both tasks, and smoothly led into a discussion of the proper performance of these procedures. The speaker was politely dismissed, a full report made to the head of respiratory therapy, and a new speaker recruited.

Charting Practice

One recurring problem in nursing orientation is the difficulty of teaching orientees how to use the different charting forms. Although instructors dutifully cover each form, explaining in great detail how it should be used, invariably complaints from the units occur: "She can't chart," "He acts as if he's never seen the discharge form before." This kind of frustration leads to hard feelings all around, with the nursing staff wondering whether anything is covered in class and the orientation instructors convinced that no one listens anymore. Of course the information is covered, and of course the orientees listen. But detailed information such as correct charting technique is not remembered by listening—only by doing.

One way to increase retention is by providing periodic practice sessions. After basic information on the appropriate forms has been covered, have orientees actually use the forms in class. Simulations are an ideal technique for achieving familiarity and confidence. Exhibit 8–8 describes a class session devoted to practice in admitting a patient. In this 45-minute segment, a videotape of an admission interview is shown. Participants then put themselves in the role of the interviewing nurse and fill out the admissions sheet, do admission charting, and begin a care plan for the patient.

Exhibit 8–8 Example of Charting Practice Class

Charting Practice Session (Admissions)

Objectives

By the end of the session the participant will be able to:

1. Completely document an admission on the Admission Sheet, leaving no blank spaces on the form.
2. Write an admitting note on the Nurses' Clinical Record; including a reason for admission, a brief systems assessment, and documentation of any identified problems.
3. Begin a nursing care plan for the admitted patient, listing at least two problems and the nursing orders related to them.

Class content

I. Provide each participant with an Admitting Sheet/Nurses' Clinical Record form and a care plan form.
II. Show Admission videotape.
III. Each participant will complete the three objectives of the session (above), using the information given in the videotape.
   A. Instructor circulates around to answer questions.
   B. When finished, get together in groups to share results and solicit peer suggestions.

Source: Education Department, Huntington Memorial Hospital, Pasadena, California. Reprinted with permission.

Another example of this approach is provided in Exhibit 8–9. In this session the participants must judge what assessment is appropriate for each patient, document their actions, and update the care plan to reflect their nursing interventions. One of the fictional patients is described in Exhibit 8–10 (the other two appeared in Exhibit 4–3 in Chapter 4). Based on the information given, which is about as much as would be obtained during nursing rounds, the nurse must decide the next steps to take. This approach not only provides an opportunity to note the orientees' skills at making judgments and charting, it also reveals how many of them identify this particular problem as a potentially lethal reaction to chloramphenicol.

In both examples, note that orientees discuss the case and get feedback from the other members of the group rather than the instructor. Naturally, the instructor should clarify information and answer questions if necessary, but on the units nurses share patient data and their ideas about it with their staff colleagues, not with an instructor. Encouraging this interaction in orientation may facilitate its happening later in actual practice.

Exhibit 8–9 Example of Charting Practice Class

Charting Practice Session (Assessment)

Objectives

By the end of the session the participant will be able to:

1. Decide what assessment steps would be appropriate for each of three patients based on a single patient contact.
2. Document the assessment you would make and any actions you would take (in the Nurses' Clinical Record).
3. Make a problem/action entry in each patient's care plan based on your judgment of the situation.

Class Content

I. Provide each participant with a care plan and a Nurses' Clinical Record.
II. Pass out the three patient cases.
III. After reading each case, the participants:
   A. Decide what assessment of the patient they will make.
      1. Write the results of their assessment (imagined results) and the actions they took.
      2. Write a care plan entry for each patient.
   B. When finished, get together in groups to share results and solicit peer suggestions.

Source: Education Department, Huntington Memorial Hospital, Pasadena, California. Reprinted with permission.

Exhibit 8–10 Patient Case from Class in Exhibit 8–9

Dave D. is a 56-year-old admitted for treatment of hypertension. He is on an 1800 calorie ADA diet (has been diabetic for ten years) and is allowed up with help. When admitted, it was noticed that he had an infected ulcer on his right ankle, which is being treated with antibiotics and wet-to-dry soaks. This morning he complained of feeling ''weak'' and of having a sore throat. When you go in to the room to assess him, you notice scattered petechiae over his trunk. His V.S. are: T. 98, P. 64, R. 20, B/P 128/88.

His drug regimen includes:
Hygroton 50 mg. daily
Inderal 40 mg. p.o. a.c. and H.S.
Chloramphenicol 250 mg. p.o. every 6 hrs.
NPH insulin 40 units subq every A.M.
ASA gr. X p.o. every 3 hrs. PRN

Other Approaches

Some other strategies that have proved useful in orientation classes include the use of skits, games, and skill laboratories.

Skits

Although most skits are brief presentations within certain classes, in at least one institution almost the entire orientation process is handled via skits. The educators have divided needed topics into three groups: (1) those that could be presented in a simulated experience, (2) those that could be covered on the unit, and (3) optional information that could wait until orientees feel a need to know it.[8] Skits involving medical, surgical, and emergency situations are outlined to incorporate all information from the first category, including policies, procedures, forms, and care routines. The actors are all staff members cast in their normal roles. Only patients and family are scripted in order to maintain spontaneity. This innovative method of presenting orientation has received positive feedback from orientees and staff alike.[9]

Gaming

There are many ways that gaming can be made a part of nursing orientation. One example was shown in Chapter 4 (see Exhibit 4–4): "Beat the Clock" is a simple game where the learner tries to complete a certain task in the least possible amount of time. In a more complicated format there may be competition between participants. (This interactive gaming must be handled carefully to prevent hard feelings.) An example is seen in Exhibit 8–11.

As with any teaching technique, gaming should be used only if it will accomplish learning objectives. In the case of the Disaster Game, participants learn important information about nursing response in a disaster by actually imagining themselves in the situation. Through study of the hospital disaster manual, orientees familiarize themselves with the hospitalwide disaster plan and project their own responses. With a large group, teams can be formed. In any case, the discussion and debriefing that occurs during and after the game provide valuable learning—far more valuable than a dry review of the hospital disaster plan.

Skills Laboratories

In one institution both learning and testing take place in a skills laboratory. During the first week of orientation, every orientee attends a lab to learn and be tested on four nursing skills: changing an IV bottle, giving an intramuscular injection, measuring urine specific gravity, and irrigating a nasogastric tube. These particular skills were chosen because instructors identified them as the ones

Exhibit 8–11 Game with Competition between Players

Disaster Game

Scenario: An earthquake is about to hit this area. It will be approximately 8.3 on the Richter Scale.

1. Roll dice to determine month of the year (1 = Jan, 2 = Feb, etc).
2. Roll one die to determine day of the week (1 = Mon, 2 = Tue, etc).
3. Roll dice to determine time of day. After a number is obtained, the instructor flips a coin: heads = A.M., tails = P.M.
4. All participants draw a card to learn where they are when the earthquake strikes (draw one card from LOCATION stack).
5. Each participant then writes on her/his tablet what she/he would do *first* during the quake. Participants take turns reading their actions aloud. As they read, the instructor tells them the results of their actions and determines their point scores.
6. As the action continues, players will be told to draw a CHANCE card periodically and read it aloud, reacting accordingly.
7. Each action must be written down and read aloud.
8. Scoring:
   a. 2 points for each appropriate action
   b. 1 point if action is partially correct
   c. 0 if action will cause no harm, even though it is inappropriate
   d. −1 if action is potentially dangerous
9. The winner is the player with the most points when outside help arrives or there are no more CHANCE cards.
10. The instructor will make the final judgment as to the usefulness of each action, but discussion from the group is welcomed.

Equipment

Coin
One pair dice
20 LOCATION cards
Tablets
Pencils
Scorecards
CHANCE cards
(21 In-hospital ones and 14 At-home ones)

Source: Reprinted from "Scenario for Disaster" by Ann Haggard, with permission of *RN Magazine*, © 1984.

most frequently lacking in orientees, as well as being necessary for daily patient care.[10]

A skills laboratory can be used only for testing, only for teaching and self-study, or in combination of all three. Skills could include any important to your hospital's practice. Many hospitals employ this approach for new graduates only, but the instructors in the example mentioned before found that all nurses should be tested, since there was no way to predict any individual's success by either experience or self-ratings.[11] Whatever way the skills laboratory is used, initial expense is high, since manikins and equipment must be purchased.

COMPETENCY-BASED ORIENTATION

An alternative to traditional, classroom-based orientation, competency-based programs require orientees to demonstrate their mastery of performance objectives within an agreed-on time frame. The knowledge required may be obtained through self-study modules, reading, discussion, or clinical practice. Hospitals using this type of program find that eliminating unnecessary class time saves money, and tailoring orientation to each person's individual needs reduces total orientation hours and increases job satisfaction.[12]

Program Design

Andragogy places great emphasis on the involvement of adult learners in a process of *self-diagnosis* of learning needs. This process consists of three phases:

1. Selecting the competencies required to achieve a given ideal model of performance.
2. Providing diagnostic experiences in which the learner can assess present competencies in light of those portrayed in the model.
3. Helping the learner measure gaps between present competencies and those required by the model, and providing educational opportunities from which the learner can select ways to bridge the gaps.[13]

Competency-based orientation programs follow this process by presenting very specific objectives that each orientee must meet. Individually, the nurses assess their present abilities to meet each criterion (through skills inventories, pretests, and discussion), and then select strategies for developing the needed skills or knowledge. This basic model is true self-directed learning.

In 1977, the American Nurses Association Ad Hoc Committee on Nontraditional Learning defined self-directed learning as "an activity for which the learner takes the initiative and responsibility for the learning process."[14] This definition supports the concept of competency-based orientation programs as a method of individual assessment and selection of learning experiences. In actual practice, though, not all orientees are capable of the self-directed approach.[15] The initial assessment determines how much help and direction each person will need from instructors and unit personnel.

Competency-Based Objectives

DelBueno, Barker, and Christmyer feel that "traditional objectives emphasize knowledge acquisition while the competency-based program emphasizes the use of knowledge in achieving competency."[16] Competencies are defined as "the technical skills, subject matter, and nursing process (judgment) that must be known and/or mastered to ensure safe patient care."[17] A comparison of traditional objectives and competency-based ones may be seen in Exhibit 8–12.

Competency-based objectives are based on performance expectations for a position. The institution might have overall competencies required of all nurses and individual unit competencies or separate service requirements (for obstetrics, critical care, orthopedics, etc.).

Developing a Learning Contract

The orientation agreement is developed along the lines of the objectives. It states all the experiences a nurse should complete before proceeding to permanent assignment. In the first meeting with an orientee, the head nurse or instructor explains the contract and negotiates the plan for meeting it. Boyer found that such a contract serves two purposes: (1) the new nurse knows exactly what is expected and (2) the instructor can pinpoint the learner's weaknesses for later follow-up and evaluation.[18]

The learning contract also provides needed structure. Douglass and Bevis found that it is essential for a learner's independence and creativity to provide some sense of the parameters of the environment (time constraints and learning aids available) and of individual learning needs (the value of knowing certain things).[19] Orientees who have difficulty diagnosing their own needs and taking responsibility for meeting them find such structure particularly helpful.

Exhibit 8–12 Traditional and Competency-Based Objectives

Traditional

The nurse will document food intake of all patients cared for, including percent eaten and how tolerated, using correct charting procedures.

Competency-based

The nurse will assess each patient's ability to select, ingest, and digest food, intervening as necessary to maintain optimum nutrition and prevent or correct eating disorders or digestive problems.

Learning Strategies

The key concepts of competency-based education may be listed as follows

1. Performance itself is the outcome.
2. Learning is self-directed with reasonable time limits.
3. Learning is self-paced to accommodate individual learning rates.
4. The teacher becomes resource rather than merely a conveyor of information.[20]

Following these principles, orientees should select their own patient assignments, and both study time and clinical time should be flexible. This can cause problems on the units if head nurses and staff are not knowledgeable and supportive of the concept. Since some content will be taught at the bedside, clinical practice must be excellent, with all nurses serving as potential role models.

Aside from planned experiences with patient care, orientees may obtain needed content from prepared learning modules. Each module usually has the following elements:

1. Title
2. Purpose statement
3. Entry behaviors
4. Objectives
5. Learning activities
6. A method of evaluation[21]

For instance, a learning module could be designed to inform learners about competency-based orientation. Exhibit 8–13 shows what the module might contain.

Learning modules can be designed to cover a wide range of content. With the addition of equipment and step-by-step procedures, orientees can even learn and practice nursing skills such as setting up for a lumbar puncture, changing ostomy bags, or instituting heart monitoring. Testing and evaluation can involve written tests, oral explanations, return demonstrations, and performance of the skill in a clinical setting.

The Instructor's Role

Orientation instructors find that competency-based programs free them from repetitive classroom instruction so they can identify and help meet individual learning needs. As the instructor role changes from teacher to learning facilitator, time can be devoted to counseling and evaluation. Although setting up learning

Exhibit 8–13 Competency-Based Orientation Module

Purpose statement: This learning module is designed to introduce the learners to the concept of competency-based orientation.

Entry behaviors: Learners should be familiar with at least one traditional orientation program, and should have participated either as instructor or preceptor.

Objectives:

1. State at least two advantages to competency-based orientation.
2. Define self-directed learning.
3. Differentiate between traditional objectives and competency-based objectives.
4. Define competencies.
5. List what a learning contract should include and the advantages of using such a contract.
6. List the four key concepts of competency-based orientation.
7. List the six elements contained in a learning module.
8. Explain at least two ways the role of the instructor is different in competency-based orientation.

Learning activities:

1. Take the pretest and score it using the key located beneath the green sheet.
2. Watch the slide/sound program by turning on the machine and pressing PLAY. Take notes using the Programmed Notes outline.
3. Test your comprehension of the material by answering the objectives for the session.
4. Listen to the audiotape "How to Develop Learning Modules," and write down the classes you feel could be converted to self-study in your situation.
5. Optional: Read the articles and/or books for additional information on the topic.
6. Take the post-test and turn it in.

Method of Evaluation:

1. Post-test scores.
2. Use of information in final assessment and practice.

modules is initially very time consuming, once the program is implemented the packages can be used over and over again with little additional revision. In the first five months of the competency-based program at Maryland General Hospital in Baltimore, both instructor time and learner time spent in orientation dropped drastically—and 90 percent of instructor time was spent in the clinical area helping the nurse apply classroom knowledge to the real world of patient care.[22]

Shaffer, Indorato, and Deneselya feel that one of the most important reasons for utilizing self-directed learning is to give the learners a sense of personal pride in their accomplishments.[23] One vital task for instructors is to help orientees recognize when they are performing effectively, so that when the instructor is no longer present the nurses can obtain personal satisfaction and reinforcement. Such internal rewards are absolutely necessary in nursing, where staff may work for long periods without once being told they are doing a good job.

Evaluation of Competency-Based Orientation

Aside from the individual learner evaluation previously discussed, how may a competency-based program be assessed? Staff and learner satisfaction are of course important, and this should be revealed by evaluations at the end of the orientee's contract completion. Cost-effectiveness must be judged by comparing the number of hours spent per learner in the orientation process, as well as the number of instructor hours spent. In one setting, learner time in the traditional program was 120 hours; in the competency-based program the time ranged from 114 to 127 hours, but most time was spent in supervised clinical experience rather than in the classroom. Instructor time dropped from 38 hours in the traditional mode to 3 hours of instruction in the competency-based process.[24]

As evaluation progresses, those responsible for orientation must ask themselves how much required content can and should be assembled in learning packages. Are these approaches effective? What should be done to teach psychomotor skills such as CPR? Perhaps a combination of self-study and classroom experience would be best, or even the traditional classroom format. Not everything must—or should—be converted to self-study. Such decisions are based on learner needs, hospital policy, and educational philosophy.

DOCUMENTATION OF LEARNING

Whether you use a traditional classroom approach to orientation or are experimenting with a newer form, good progress records for each orientee are vital. Poor records result in confusion as the orientees move to their individual units. They can even result in potential legal problems later. If an orientee brings a labor board action or lawsuit against the hospital and the orientation experience is inadequately documented, the hospital has lost the case. To prevent this, as well as to forestall numerous phone calls during orientation from puzzled orientees and irate head nurses, document each area of content covered.

Exhibit 8–14 provides an example of one such record form. As each segment is completed, the instructor and the orientee initial in the appropriate space to show that the information has been presented. On the unit the clinician, preceptor, or head nurse validate its application to clinical practice or instruction. The space allowed for progress notes allows the classroom instructor to record the orientee's attitude toward learning, ability to grasp concepts, and any other information important for the unit to know. Since this form will be a permanent part of the employee's record and may be referred to during evaluation sessions, such

Exhibit 8–14 Sample Documentation Form

R.N./L.V.N. ORIENTATION CHECKLIST

EMPLOYEE ______________________ ORIENTATION START DATE __________

TOPICS	INSTRUCTOR DATE/INITIALS	CLINICIAN DATE/INITIALS	EMPLOYEE DATE/INITIALS
I. GENERAL INFORMATION			
Hospital Philosophy			
Organization Structure			
Benefits			
Job Description			
Badge In/Badge Out			
Exception Reports			
Sick Calls			
Employee Policies			
Professional Liability			
II. NURSING UNIT			
Physical Layout			
Location of equipment/supplies			
Methods of assignment			
Time schedules			
Special requests			
Shift change reporting system			
Charting guidelines			
Kardex			
Discharge planning			
Pneumatic tube system			
Evaluations			

III. PATIENT CARE REPORTS Patient Charts			
Notification forms			
Medication Error Reports			
Responsibility releases			
Patient census/condition reports			
Discharge sheet			
Decubitus care form			
Code Blue report forms			
Surgery consent forms			
Pre-operative checklists			

IV. POLICIES/PROCEDURES Admissions			
Transfers			
Discharges			
Surgery (pre & post-operative care)			
Death			
Intake/Output			
Isolation/Infection Control			
Transcribing Physician Orders			
Blood Transfusions			
IV Therapy			
Medication Administration			
Narcotic Control			
Fire Procedure			
Evacuation/Disasters			
Code Blue Procedures			
Nursing Care Plans			
Suctioning			
Oxygen Administration			
Op-site/stomadhesive			
Feeding tubes			
Electrical Safety			

Exhibit 8–14 continued

PROGRESS NOTES: ______________________________

____

____

____

____

____

____

____

INSTRUCTOR: ____________ CLINICIAN: ____________ EMPLOYEE: ____________

documentation should be based on fact and defensible. Recording anecdotal notes about observable behavior will prevent subjective opinion from creeping in.

CONCLUSION

The initial classroom work in nursing orientation is geared to provide orientees with the information they need to give safe, effective patient care. Whether traditional learning methods or self-directed study are employed, this learning must be carefully planned and validated by the orientation instructor.

In Chapter 9 clinical orientation will be discussed, with special emphasis on the role of the unit preceptor. Although all of orientation is important, what happens in the work setting has the most immediate impact on new employees. How clinical orientation is handled will have a profound effect on their careers not only with the institution but even with the entire profession of nursing.

NOTES

1. *Accreditation Manual for Hospitals, 1983 Edition* (Chicago: Joint Commission on Accreditation of Hospitals, 1983), 120.

2. Christine Fredericks, "Reversing the Turnover Trend," *Nursing Management* 12, no. 12 (December 1981): 42.

3. Helen M. Tobin, Pat S. Yoder-Wise, and Peggy K. Hull, *The Process of Staff Development: Components for Change*, 2d ed. (St. Louis: C.V. Mosby Co., 1979), 119.

4. Marjorie Moore Cantor, "Who Decides and Who Is Accountable?" *Journal of Nursing Administration* 6, no. 3 (May-June 1974), 23.

5. Ascher J. Segall et al., *Systematic Course Design for the Health Fields* (New York: John Wiley and Sons, 1975), A–66.

6. Martin M. Broadwell, *The Supervisor As an Instructor: A Guide for Classroom Training*, 2d ed. (Reading, Mass.: Addison-Wesley Publishing Co., 1970), 151.

7. Marjorie Moore Cantor, "Education for Quality Care," *Journal of Nursing Administration* 5, no. 1 (January-February 1973): 11.

8. Patricia Reagan, "Orientation the Off-Off Broadway Way," *American Journal of Nursing* 73, no. 7 (July 1973): 1223.

9. Ibid., 1224.

10. Martha Schmidt Kaelin and Julie Beshore Bliss, "Evaluating Newly Employed Nurses' Skills," *Nursing Outlook* 27, no. 5 (May 1979): 334.

11. Ibid., 336.

12. Margaret D. Sovie, "The Role of Staff Development in Hospital Cost Control," *Nurse Educator* 5, no. 6 (November-December 1980): 27.

13. Malcolm S. Knowles, *The Modern Practice of Adult Education* (Chicago: Association Press, Follett Publishing Co., 1980), 47–48.

14. Deanne F. Bell and Durward L. Bell, "Harmonizing Self-Directed and Teacher-Directed Approaches to Learning," *Nurse Educator* 8, no. 1 (Spring 1983): 24.

15. Tobin, Yoder-Wise, and Hull, *The Process of Staff Development,* 150.

16. Dorothy J. delBueno, Frances Barker, and Carol Christmyer, ''Implementing a Competency-Based Orientation Program,'' *Nurse Educator* 5, no. 3 (May-June 1980): 16.

17. Sharon Ghiglieri, Susan Ann Woods, and Kerry Moyer, ''Toward a Competency-Based Safe Practice,'' *Nursing Management* 14, no. 3 (March 1983): 17.

18. Catherine Boyer, ''Performance-Based Staff Development: The Cost-Effective Alternative,'' *Nurse Educator* 6, no. 5 (September-October 1981): 13.

19. Laura Mae Douglass and Em Olivia Bevis, *Nursing Leadership in Action* (St. Louis: C.V. Mosby Co., 1974), 45.

20. Ghiglieri, Woods, and Moyer, ''Toward a Competency-Based Safe Practice,'' 16.

21. Bell and Bell, ''Self-Directed and Teacher-Directed Approaches,'' 25.

22. delBueno, Barker, and Christmyer, ''Implementing a Competency-Based Program,'' 27.

23. Stuart M. Shaffer, Karen L. Indorato, and Janet A. Deneselya, *Teaching in Schools of Nursing* (St. Louis: C.V. Mosby Co., 1972), 42.

24. delBueno, Barker, and Christmyer, ''Implementing a Competency-Based Program,'' 27.

Chapter 9

Orientation in the Clinical Area

However outstanding the orientation classes may be, it is in the clinical area that orientees are either made or broken. Unfortunately, all too often orientation is not a high priority, and new employees become victims of a functional "get the nine o'clocks passed" approach. This is doubly unfortunate because it not only hurts the orientees, but boomerangs on the unit staff, who will be doomed to a constant flow of new people to orient as turnover takes its toll. Since staff instability is one of the causes of poor unit orientation, a vicious cycle is established that is hard to break.

If your institution has no formal plan for orienting new nurses once they reach the clinical area, or if you think that the existing plan needs revision, propose a task force to examine the problem. Since unit staff will be handling the crucial parts of orientation, nurses from the various units should be on the task force. The tasks of this group involve the following:

1. Identifying the problem
2. Analyzing the causes of the problem
3. Finding practical solutions
4. Developing and implementing a plan for putting these solutions to work, including methods of evaluation.

ANALYZING CLINICAL ORIENTATION

The Problem

Tobin, Yoder-Wise, and Hull state that "regardless of past experience, new employees need opportunities to practice in the new environment."[1] The key word is *practice*. *Webster's Third New International Dictionary* defines it as "to exercise oneself in for instruction or improvement or for the acquisition of discipline, proficiency, or dexterity," and secondarily "to exercise another in something for similar purposes."[2] Practice implies a period of learning and supervised experience.

Why then are so many orientees given a quick tour of the unit (if they receive that) and then handed a full patient assignment with the words "I know you can handle this," or "I think people learn best by just diving right in, don't you?" Chances are the orientee will manage to complete the assignment, but at what cost to self-esteem and adrenalin?

A planned orientation is designed to achieve optimum employee effectiveness in the least time possible. Rather than "turn them loose" and allow orientees to stumble blindly in search of their roles, save time and money by providing guidance and support. Merrill found that a planned, organized and meaningful orientation is critical to nurses' performance and job satisfaction and ultimately to staff retention.[3]

Causes of the Problem

Why are so many orientees shortchanged in the clinical area? The list of reasons may include:

1. Rapid turnover in staff
2. Understaffing
3. Head nurse and staff not seeing orientation as a priority
4. Too many orientees at one time
5. Lack of support from administration
6. An attitude of "I lived through it—so can they"
7. Lack of an organized plan for orienting new people

In your setting you might find some, all, or none of these conditions. You may also come up with completely different reasons for the problem. But once the causes have been identified, scrutinize them carefully. Are the units really understaffed, or is that just a rote complaint trotted out to explain every nursing problem? What hard data can you find to support the conclusion (nurse-patient ratios, patient classification requirements, comparisons with other hospitals)? Such analysis of the causes prevents an automatic reaction of "It's always been that way and nothing will change it." Has it always been that way? What way? Why can't it be changed? Should it be changed? The people concerned with problem analysis need to take every idea and assumption and turn it upside down to be thoroughly shaken out. Think of creative new ways of looking at things.

Finding and Implementing Solutions

Once the problem nas been identified and causes analyzed, solutions can be found. If no serious organizational problems exist (such as severe understaffing), often just making people aware of the problem serves to focus attention on it and create solutions. Such solutions may be both organizational and educational, but ultimately they will lead to an organized plan for orienting new employees.

Each unit's approach to orientation must be arrived at by the staff involved. What experiences did they have as orientees? What proved helpful? What was upsetting? What can they do to ease new people into the group in a way that will make orientees want to stay and contribute to the unit? Brainstorming sessions help lead to strategies each work group can implement to orient new nurses in the most effective way.

The first six months of any newly hired nurse's employment is the most critical period—and the word *any* should be stressed. Weisman et al. found that the process of job acclimation was the same for both new graduates and experienced nurses.[4] Adjustment to the organization seemed to be more important than role transition, with the nature of the work environment determining job satisfaction and eventual turnover.[5] These findings imply that orientation for all nurses, no matter what their experience, should focus on familiarizing them with the particular organizational factors that affect performance.

STRATEGIES FOR CLINICAL ORIENTATION

Skills Inventories

When new employees assess their own knowledge and abilities via the skills inventory, unit personnel have a guide for planning individualized orientation. Exhibit 9–1 shows a portion of such an inventory completed by an orientee. Using it as a guide, unit people (head nurse, clinician, preceptor) can meet with the new person to mutually plan ways of providing experiences needed. Follow-up is crucially important. The orientee must not only have the opportunity to perform the procedure, performance must be observed and validated, with feedback given on safety and effectiveness.

One way that the use of the skills inventory can be expanded is through a performance checklist. This lists each behavior required to successfully perform procedures, differentiating them as "critical" or "desired." The new nurse must demonstrate all critical behaviors for successful completion.[6] A criterion-referenced checklist of this sort can also be used for objective task evaluation of orientees.

Exhibit 9–1 Excerpt from Completed Skills Inventory

Task Performance	A	B	C	Comments
3. Suction equipment				
A. Gomco	X			
B. Hi-Low	X			
C. Wall				
1. Oral	X			
2. Suct. Inter.	X			
D. Hemovac	X			
E. Pleur-Evac		X		Don't feel confident
4. Insertion/Removal of				
A. Levin tube		X		Would like supervision
B. Foley catheter	X			
C. Straight catheter			X	Never done
5. Collection of				
A. Sterile specimen		X		Done once
B. Clean catch	X			
C. Clinitest/Acetest	X			
D. Testape	X			
E. Specific gravity	X			
F. 24 hour urine	X			
G. Straining for stones	X			
H. Sputum--AFB	X			
I. Gastric contents			X	Never seen

The First Day on the Unit

The first day on the unit may come the very first day of employment for some, and not until the beginning of the second week for others, depending on the orientation schedule. Regardless of when it happens, the first clinical day is anxiety-filled, as the new nurse strives to make a good first impression on co-workers.

At this most critical point in orientation, a planned, organized approach to learning lessens apprehension and provides greater satisfaction and security for new employees. Of course, the unit has been informed of the hiring and start date, but be sure someone is there to welcome the new person. It is disturbing to stand uncomfortably at the desk waiting for someone to acknowledge your presence.

The ideal person to greet the newcomer is the head nurse. To staff nurses, their head nurse *is* the hospital, symbolizing the entire organization through the power to reward and discipline. Studies have shown that the single most important factor affecting the productivity and satisfaction of nurses is the head nurse.[7] Considering this impact, a welcome from the manager is a good way to start the first day.

Since managers are ultimately responsible for orientation and its results, the head nurse should sit down and discuss the unit and the orientee's personal objectives as a nurse. This initial meeting serves to clear up misconceptions about the role of a nurse on this particular unit, and to clarify expectations about scheduling, performance, autonomy, etc., on the parts of both head nurse and orientee.

Should the orientee have a patient assignment on the first day? The purpose of assignments during orientation is to help new nurses learn where things are, how the care system works, and what their responsibilities are. If orientees are given a few patients and told "Ask me if you have any questions," how is learning to occur? The new nurse will open a lot of drawers and cabinets to locate needed equipment, try to learn the system by observation and timid questions, and explore responsibilities by trial and error. Learning by making mistakes is ineffective and inefficient. If new people don't receive instruction and guidance, their first assignments will be unsatisfactory. Frohman found that the results of poor first assignments are excessive start-up time and poor mastery of the job.[8]

Another approach to the first day is to have the new person walk around the unit, observe all the staff, and read manuals. If you have ever spent an entire day observing and reading manuals, then you know it is an exhausting, boring way to use your time, and the learning that occurs is limited. New employees want to be doing things, experiencing their new roles in a real and practical way.

So what can orientees do on the first day? To strike a happy medium between making the orientees completely responsible for patients and making them wander around the unit with little to do, use the buddy system. Each orientee is paired with an experienced staff nurse. On the first day, the staff nurse receives a patient assignment—not heavier than usual; if anything, a little lighter—and the orientee works with the buddy to care for these patients. Notice that the orientee is not assigned any patients. The whole purpose of this method of orientation is that the new person works alongside the experienced nurse to learn care routines. If one is in one room giving a bath while the other is down the hall passing medications, all the benefits of the buddy system are lost.

As the new nurse becomes more comfortable on the unit, separate assignments are made, with the buddy still available as a resource. If possible, the pair should be scheduled for the same on-duty time through the end of the orientation period. The buddy system of orientation is based on the adult education principle that a role model shapes a learner's behavior by narrowing the range of acceptable behavior through a system of social reward and punishment.[9] Later in the chapter the use of preceptors will be discussed, an approach that takes the buddy system one step further.

METHODS OF CLINICAL INSTRUCTION

Once on the unit, most orientee learning happens as a result of one-on-one instruction. Whether this is done by the head nurse, orientation instructor, unit clinician, assigned buddy, or whoever happens to be around, how it is done can have a significant impact on the orientee's self-confidence and attitude toward the unit. Ideally, whoever instructs new people should have a vested interest in helping them do well, as managers, instructors, and assigned unit teachers do. The danger of having whoever's handy answer questions or demonstrate procedures is that "whoever's handy" may be a poor instructor, give wrong information, be angry or impatient, or even deliberately lead the new employee astray. Merrill found that a person who does not like to orient new people or who practices with only minimal proficiency can negate all previous preparation.[10]

Using the skills inventory or performance checklist as a guide, the person responsible for unit instruction can plan the sequence of clinical orientation. After assessing the orientee's educational background, past experience, and anxiety level, discuss how he or she learns best: explanation, demonstration, reading, performing the procedure with feedback? The approach to teaching the procedures and routines of care will vary according to orientee learning style, instructor teaching style, and time available.

Analysis of Instruction

Certain problems arise again and again in clinical instruction. Some of these include:

1. Assuming background knowledge that is not there
2. Failing to organize instruction in a logical way
3. Failing to set objectives
4. Inadequate testing and follow-up

All of these problems are preventable. Discussion of the skills inventory with the orientee should clear up any questions about background knowledge and experience. Objectives must always be set for the learner, which almost automatically organizes instruction logically. If head nurses and preceptors have difficulty with the idea of writing objectives, provide assistance. This may involve teaching them how to write objectives or even providing prepared objectives. Exhibit 9–2 shows an excerpt from some clinical objectives for orientees that provide needed guidance and organization. Naturally, these can be changed or renegotiated by the head nurse and preceptor.

Testing and follow-up are an ongoing part of clinical orientation. Through observation, questioning, conferences, and examination of charting, care plans, and other forms of documentation, the person responsible for orientation validates the orientee's performance. Note in Exhibit 9–2 that the last objective on Friday forces sharing of results and goals. If nursing care standards are clearly communicated and mistakes or misunderstandings corrected immediately, new nurses should quickly discover how to perform up to unit expectations.

Patient Assignments for Instruction

Too often the orientees are assigned patients according to room numbers. Automatically giving the nurse "Rooms 20 through 25" ignores the employee's learning needs and the patients' care needs. What experiences are needed by the orientee? What patient needs could best be met by this person? During orientation assignments should be used as learning tools.

The best way to determine assignments is to ask the orientee to choose the patients most likely to provide needed experience. Each experience should reinforce and build on previous ones, so maintain planned assignments for new employees. For instance, if the new nurse is learning team leading, the first step would be to buddy for at least two days with an experienced staff member. Then the orientee leads a team of perhaps eight patients. This gives time to work problems through slowly, so the novice team leader can get a handle on institutional forms and routines. Gradually increase the number of patients until the orientee is carrying a full team. This is not a strategy just for new graduates—it should be done for experienced nurses as well, to enable them to adjust their approach from old ways of performing to your institution's methods.

Another important point about assignments: don't assign new employees to off shifts or weekends until they are comfortable with the unit. When orientees work

Exhibit 9–2 Clinical Objectives

Second Week

Wednesday, 7–3:30 on unit.

While working with the unit secretary and charge nurse:

1. Practice all CRT functions learned in class until accurate and complete.
2. Transcribe at least six sets of physician's orders, having them checked by the charge nurse before entering into system.
3. Use the CRT manuals for other departments to become familiar with their layout and capabilities.
4. Observe how standard care plans are selected and used.
5. Note the use of the daily patient information sheet, daily diet report, and day/night report.
6. Complete the manual self-study and observe how information contained in the manuals is used to help with decisions/actions of the staff.

Thursday, 7–3:30 on unit.

While working alone, with preceptor as backup:

1. Take report on assigned patients, checking with preceptor about any questions or ambiguities.
2. Give total patient care to three patients, including: AM care, help with meals, bath and bedmaking, medications, ambulation, treatments, patient/family teaching, care plans, and charting.
3. Work with clinician/head nurse to obtain any additional information necessary.
4. Give report on your patients to oncoming shift.

Friday, 7–3:30 on unit.

While working alone, with preceptor as backup:

1. Complete objectives 1 through 4 from Thursday with an assignment of four patients.
2. Perform the complete admission procedure with at least one patient, including beginning the nursing care plan.
3. Help with at least one patient discharge.
4. Review the location of other departments your unit uses or goes to frequently, such as satellite pharmacy or blood bank.
5. Talk to the head nurse about the following: your use of care plans, your charting, your plans and goals as a nurse and how they will fit into unit plans and goals.

at a sparsely staffed time they may not have the help and support they need to operate effectively. Poor performance is devastating to everyone. Spare orientees by establishing criteria that all staff members must meet before being assigned to evenings, nights, or weekends.

Effect of Instructor Behaviors

O'Shea conducted a study in a nursing program that identified teaching behaviors that facilitate learning in the clinical setting as well as those that interfere with learning. A number of facilitative behaviors were identified:

1. Being willing to help
2. Answering questions freely
3. Demonstrating and explaining new procedures
4. Assisting with problems
5. Giving honest feedback
6. Being supportive, friendly, and enthusiastic[11]

The negative behaviors included:

1. Having unrealistic expectations
2. Not recognizing individual differences
3. Giving insufficient or only negative feedback
4. Lack of clearly defined expectations
5. Authoritarian or intimidating manner
6. Criticizing in the presence of others
7. Being impersonal or condescending[12]

Off-Unit Observation

Many hospitals include a series of observations in other departments. The advantage of this relates to fostering identification with the hospital as a whole and learning how other areas contribute to patient care. Meeting people from other units and seeing how they function leads to better communication later on. The disadvantage is that such observation pulls orientees away from their own work groups, disrupting the socialization process so vital to good work relations. These observations can also add to information overload for the new employees, crowding out more important data about their own unit and their practice of nursing in that setting.

The best way to decide whether to send orientees in your institution for off-unit observation is to examine the objectives of orientation. Will such observation help the new employees achieve personal or program objectives better than working on the home unit? If not, the off-unit time should be converted to planned patient care assignments and observation within the orientee's work group. Unless you can demonstrate that observations in other departments contribute in some measurable way to the new person's ultimate success, the off-unit experience falls into the "nice-to-know" category and should be dropped from the program.

Use of Orientation Units

Placing orientees on units designated expressly for orientation is a practice seen in some hospitals. The rationale for this approach is that the entire unit is geared toward teaching and there is more supervision available. On some of these units the staff provides the instruction; on others the orientation instructors from the education department work with orientees.

These units are set up by meeting with staff to explore their feelings about orientation and to secure their support for the concept. Plans are made for assigning all new nurses to the orientation unit(s) for a designated period of time, usually the first two weeks of employment. When a nurse is hired, all clinical experience is provided on the special unit. At the end of the orientation unit assignment, the nurse moves to the permanent work area.

Although the instruction received on such a unit is well planned and well executed, several serious drawbacks exist. First, the orientees are placed in an artificial environment that some may resent as being too protected and too much like a student experience in nursing school. Second, the staff of such a unit may rapidly burn out from a heavy influx of orientees. Instructing and supporting many new people week after week is exhausting. Third, and perhaps most important, orientees are kept from their home unit and permanent work group, delaying bonding and identification and increasing costs as they still have to be oriented to their own unit.

The decision as to whether or not to institute an orientation unit should be made as any other decision about orientation is made: by asking whether it will fulfill the program objectives. In what way will working on a special unit ease transition to the new role and facilitate effective performance and job satisfaction? What can be accomplished on such a unit that cannot be accomplished on the orientees' permanent work areas? Why? You may find it simpler and ultimately better for all concerned to concentrate planning and resources in order to improve clinical orientation on every unit rather than segregating orientees in a single special area

PRECEPTOR PROGRAMS IN CLINICAL ORIENTATION

A preceptor is an experienced nurse selected according to specific criteria to serve as a resource person to new nurses.[13] Although formal preceptor programs are a fairly new development in orientation, the concept of an experienced practitioner serving as a mentor to a new person has been around for as long as there have been trades and professions. Recently, hospitals have developed programs to prepare especially proficient staff as role models for new nurses.

These programs are expensive to start, because the preceptors must be prepared for their new role. After the initial cost outlay, however, this approach to orientation can pay for itself in increased staff effectiveness and decreased turnover.

Selecting Preceptors

The selection of staff nurses to serve as preceptors is usually done by the head nurses. The people selected should be volunteers, but not all volunteers are appropriate choices. Criteria for selection include:

1. At least one year's experience in the clinical area
2. Permanent, full-time employee
3. Consistent high-quality nursing skills and judgment
4. Desire to work closely with new employees
5. Ability to instruct others clearly and in a positive, supportive way

Benefits of the position include increased status and the opportunity to practice teaching skills as well as bedside care. Many programs also add monetary rewards. In one hospital, preceptors receive a 10 percent increase in pay to compensate for the added responsibility of the position, as well as having five conference days per year to perform job-related duties.[14]

Preceptor Preparation

After the nurses have been selected, preparation for their new role should include a workshop and discussion meetings. The workshop should be a minimum of one day in length if the preceptors are to have a basic grounding in what they will be doing. The best way to introduce the subject is to ask the group what a preceptor is and does. Write down all the responses and take off from there into a discussion of roles, responsibilities, and opportunities. A wonderful quote can be used at this point: Lucie Young Kelly once stated that no matter what direction nurses' careers take, "somewhere they have to learn the ropes, sense the political climate, spot the behind-the-scenes action, gain insights into the field, and have a sounding board for decisions."[15] What better description of the preceptor role could there be?

Specific areas of content for the workshop include:

1. Adult education principles
2. Methods of learning needs assessment
3. How to formulate specific written objectives
4. Methods of clinical instruction
5. The role of a role model
6. How to give and receive feedback
7. Counseling and evaluating new employees

Although preceptors need the didactic information on these subjects, be sure to provide practical experience as well. Have them assess their own learning styles, identify assessment methods they can use on the unit, write objectives, plan and practice at least one new teaching method, and role play giving feedback and counseling to each other. Further needs of the preceptors can be discovered during the initial workshop, and ways to meet them devised—follow-up classes, resources for self-study, rap sessions for all members, or individual counseling.

Each preceptor should meet with the head nurse to determine how orientation will be conducted on the unit. Will the unit have only one preceptor, or one for each shift? If only one, will that person rotate to the other shifts with orientees? If not, who will be responsible for teaching and supporting new people on evenings and nights? Everyone must be clear on what will be happening—and consensus should be reached about it. If there is disagreement or dissatisfaction with the plan, such problems should be discussed and settled before an orientee gets caught in the middle.

Implementing the Preceptor Program

Ideally, preceptors meet orientees on the first day of orientation, perhaps at the luncheon during the new employee orientation. A formal meeting takes place on the first clinical day, when the preceptor greets the new person on arrival to the unit and initiates the mentor relationship. Exhibit 9–3 shows guidelines for the different roles involved in orientation: head nurse, preceptor, educator, and new employee.

Murphy and Hammerstad suggest that during the first meeting on the unit, the preceptor and orientee discuss the preceptor role and agree on how much help the new nurse would like. Would the orientee prefer to observe for a short period and then plunge right in, to work together for a longer period, or some other approach?[16]

Besides working with the new nurse to demonstrate expert practice and instruct on policies and procedures, the preceptor is also responsible for easing the socialization process. One of the most valuable things a preceptor can do is cue the orientee into the norms of the work group, those unwritten rules that determine acceptance into group culture. Everson et al. found it possible for a new nurse to repeatedly violate systems expectations simply by behaving in accordance with the norms or rules of the previous system.[17] This can be avoided if the preceptor takes the time to tell the new person when behavior is acceptable and when it is in violation of unwritten rules.

Regular meetings should be scheduled to provide time for formal feedback on how orientation is progressing. Although informal feedback is exchanged almost constantly as the two nurses work together, in the meetings they examine the process rather than the outcomes. What is the preceptor doing that has proved helpful? Not helpful? Has anything come up that is causing problems? Are the goals and objectives of the orientation program and the individual being accomplished?

Evaluating the Preceptor Program

Ideally, there is no set time for each person's orientation to end when using a preceptor program. Each sequence is as individualized as the learning strategies used by the preceptors, and no deadline for completion is set. However, in many programs the end of orientation is within a certain number of weeks unless problems develop, preceptor or no preceptor. The reasons for this are practical: new orientees compete for the preceptor's time and the more experienced new employees must be counted as staff fairly quickly or costs become prohibitive.

In any individualized program of orientation, evaluation is crucial because a lack of set checkpoints makes it easy to miss important information. Preceptor programs usually build in evaluation strategies such as tests and questionnaires as well as feedback sessions and performance appraisals (see Exhibit 9–3). While these approaches will be discussed in detail in Chapter 13, the results of evaluating some preceptor programs may be of interest.

Follow-up questionnaires used in May's program indicated that all orientees found having a preceptor reduced the anticipated pressures of orientation. This was true whether the new nurse was experienced or newly graduated.[18] Preceptors and the overall support from peers were the most helpful elements in orientation, according to answers received from Patton, Grace, and Rocca's evaluation of the program; some orientees stated that preceptors were so important to their adjustment that they felt anyone oriented without such support would be at a disadvantage.[19] Atwood discovered that many staff members expressed increased job satisfaction from a preceptor program; in addition, patient questionnaires and patient and family interviews indicated that patients received better care when the practice of the more experienced nurse was extended.[20]

A final consideration when evaluating the program is preceptor burnout. When preceptors deal with one new employee after another without an occasional break, exhaustion and frustration are inevitable. The evaluation process should have some mechanism built in to identify this condition before it becomes critical. One way that may prove helpful is a regular preceptor meeting, where all preceptors join with their peers and the orientation coordinator to discuss the program and their feelings about it. Preceptors can discuss their frustrations and identify strategies to deal with such problems as trying to guide more than one new employee at a time. Plasse and Lederer discovered that burnout can be prevented or lessened by providing adequate staffing so that the preceptor has time away from patient assignments to work with the new employees.[21]

Exhibit 9–3 Roles in a Preceptor Program

	HEAD NURSE	PRECEPTOR	NURSE EDUCATOR	NEW EMPLOYEE
ASSESSMENT	1. Interviews and hires new employee with input from AHN. 2. Administers Clinical Unit Skills Inventory 3. Pretests for theory and clinical abilities 4. Compares new employee to competencies in CORE Curriculum	1. Reviews results of and explains use of: • Clinical Skills Inventory • CORE Curriculum • Objectives • Other tests given to new employee 2. Direct observation of new employee clinical performance	1. Reviews results of • Clinical Skills Inventory • CORE Curriculum • Other tests given 2. Direct observation of new employee performance	1. Completes and updates Clinical Skills Inventory self-assessment of current performance level 2. Identifies own learning needs
PLANNING	1. Selects Preceptor for new employee 2. Informs Nursing Education, Preceptor & Unit Staff of new employee's hire date and learning needs 3. Assigns new employee to orient day shift and/or off shift	1. Has planning conference with new employee first clinical day 2. Writes mutually agreed upon goals and objectives to increase skill and performance level of new employee	1. Informs Preceptor & Unit of first clinical day 2. Assists Preceptor in writing goals & objectives	1. Writes mutually agreed upon goals and objectives with Preceptor
IMPLEMENTATION	1. Provides orientation and Preceptor time for new employee	1. Is not "in charge" while Precepting 2. Provides Learning Center time for new employee 3. Provides learning activ-	1. Provides new employee with general hospital orientation 2. Provide Preceptors with Preceptor Training Program	1. Reads Procedure & Policy manuals 2. Initiates own learning experiences 3. Follows learning activ-

		ities for new employee 4. Acts as clinical resource for new employee 5. Weekly conferences to review progress on technical and process skills 6. Gives ongoing feedback regarding performance 7. Validates Skills according to Protocol	3. Assists Preceptor in locating appropriate learning activities	ities outlined in CORE Curriculum and follows "Guidelines for Integrating Nursing Process into Practice"
EVALUATION	1. Evaluates orientee's progress by observation & feedback from orientee and Preceptor 2. Conducts 3-month evaluation conference with Preceptor and new employee 3. Determines if orientation needs to be extended 4. Assigns new employee to permanent status	1. Conferences with new employees about progress at end of orientation 2. Give feedback to HN regarding new employee performance 3. Provides written evaluation to new employee using goals & objectives direct observation Clinical Unit Skills Inventory Process to Practice Tool	1. Assists Preceptor & new employee in evaluating new employee's progress 2. Consults on any proposed extension of probation or orientation 3. Evaluates orientation and updates learning programs as needed 4. Reviews orientation evaluations and gives feedback to Preceptors and Head Nurses	1. Conferences with Head Nurse and Preceptor at end of orientation 2. Evaluates Preceptor program and orientation 3. Writes self-evaluation of progress with use of Clinical Unit Skills Inventory & mutually set goals & objectives

Source: Nancy Plasse and Janet Reiss Lederer, "Preceptor: A Resource for New Nurses," *Supervisor Nurse* 12, no. 6 (June 1981): 40. Reprinted with permission of Nursing Management, © 1981.

COSTS OF CLINICAL ORIENTATION

A major reason for rushing orientees into full assignments before they are ready is a desire to keep costs down for the unit. The sooner new people can be counted on the staffing sheet, the less down-time cost. Using this philosophy results in forcing unprepared orientees into giving less than optimal care. Both patients and employees suffer. Yet it is hard to blame the unit manager, who is receiving tremendous pressure from above to control unit costs.

One solution is to designate a special cost center for orientees. When new people are hired, they are paid from this orientation cost center for at least the first two weeks. Time cards are verified and signed by the orientation coordinator. This approach transfers the costs of orienting new people off the shoulders of the head nurse. It also enables you to analyze cost-benefit ratios more exactly, since the costs are isolated from the rest of the operating budget. Fredericks found that placing new staff under a special cost center clearly distinguishes between regular staff and orientee functions and costs patterns, and helps prevent orientee overload by keeping them from being counted as staff before they are ready.[22]

CONCLUSION

Clinical orientation is the single most important aspect of bringing new employees on board in the organization. Each institution must analyze its approach to orienting new nurses to patient care and select strategies to deal with the inevitable problems. Whether a traditional system is used or a new method such as precepting tried, all staff must be involved in orienting new employees to the clinical area.

Chapter 10 will examine new graduate orientation, a subject that has come into increasing prominence in the past few years. Different approaches have been tried, with varying results, and every hospital must decide on its own program for facilitating entry to professional nursing practice. Numerous strategies for achieving this will be discussed.

NOTES

1. Helen M. Tobin, Pat S. Yoder-Wise, and Peggy K. Hull, *The Process of Staff Development: Components for Change*, 2d ed. (St. Louis: C.V. Mosby Co., 1979), 149.

2. *Webster's Third New International Dictionary of the English Language, Unabridged, 17th Edition* (Chicago: Encyclopedia Britannica, 1976), 1780.

3. Sunny Merrill, "Commitment Needed for Effective Staff Orientation Program," *AORN Journal* 34, no. 3 (September-October 1981): 379.

4. Carol S. Weisman et al., "Employment Patterns Among Newly Hired Hospital Staff Nurses: A Comparison of Nursing Graduates and Experienced Nurses," *Nursing Research* 30, no. 3 (May-June 1981): 189.

5. Ibid., 191.

6. Colleen McCaffrey, "Performance Checklists: An Effective Method of Teaching, Learning, and Evaluating," *Nurse Educator* 3, no. 1 (January-February 1978): 11.

7. Alan L. Frohman, "More Effective Development for New Nurses," *Nursing Administration Quarterly* 1, no. 2, (Summer 1977): 32–33.

8. Ibid., 39.

9. Dee Ann Gillies, *Nursing Management: A Systems Approach* (Philadelphia: W.B. Saunders Co., 1982), 211.

10. Merrill, "Commitment Needed," 380.

11. Helen Spustek O'Shea and Margaret Kidd Parsons, "Clinical Instruction: Effective and Ineffective Teacher Behaviors," *Nursing Outlook* 27, no. 6 (June 1979): 413.

12. Ibid., 414.

13. Nancy J. Plasse and Janet Reiss Lederer, "Preceptors: A Resource for New Nurses," *Supervisor Nurse* 12, no. 6 (June 1981): 35.

14. Gerald Lee and Edith D. Raleigh, "A Half-Way House for the New Graduate," *Nursing Management* 14, no. 1 (January 1983): 43.

15. Lucie Young Kelly, "Power Guide—the Mentor Relationship," *Nursing Outlook* 26, no. 5 (May 1978): 339.

16. Mary Lou Murphy and Susan M. Hammerstad, "Preparing a Staff Nurse for Precepting," *Nurse Educator* 6, no. 5 (September-October 1981): 18.

17. Sally Everson et al., "Precepting as an Entry Method for Newly Hired Staff," *The Journal of Continuing Education in Nursing* 12, no. 5 (1981): 25.

18. Louise May, "Clinical Preceptors for New Nurses," *American Journal of Nursing* 80, no. 10 (October 1980): 1826.

19. Dorothy Patton, Annette Grace, and Jean Rocca, "Implementation of the Preceptor Concepts: Adaptation to High Stress Climate," *The Journal of Continuing Education in Nursing* 12, no. 5 (1981): 30.

20. Aileen H. Atwood, "The Mentor in Clinical Practice," *Nursing Outlook* 27, no. 11 (November 1979): 717.

21. Plasse and Lederer, "Preceptors," 41.

22. Christine Fredericks, "Reversing the Turnover Trend," *Nursing Management* 12, no. 12 (December 1981): 44.

Chapter 10

New Graduate Orientation

Why do we have special orientation for nurses newly graduated from the basic preparatory programs? As late as the 1960s, such a thing was almost unknown. New graduates were hired and oriented in exactly the same way as a nurse who had worked for ten years. There was no thought of providing a special program, and neither the staff nor the new graduates themselves expected such a thing.

It was in the 1960s, however, that the seeds of change were sown. The American Nurses' Association "Position Paper on Nursing Education" was published in 1965, causing an instant uproar with its controversial recommendations that basic educational preparation in nursing should be at the university level. At the same time, the few two-year associate degree programs that began in the 1950s were coming into their own. In the years since the position paper rocked the profession, significant and lasting changes have occurred in nursing education. First, the number of baccalaureate graduates has increased greatly. Second, the number of associate degree graduates has skyrocketed as these programs continue to proliferate. And third, the number of diploma graduates who receive their basic preparation in a hospital environment has dropped drastically.

This is not the place to discuss the pros and cons of these changes; whether the changes in nursing education will be the making or the ruination of the profession has been debated at length in the literature and no doubt will continue to be debated for some time to come. What affects hospitals educators is this: these changes have produced a markedly different end product. Whether the new graduates have come from a baccalaureate, associate degree, or diploma program, they share these characteristics:

1. They have a wealth of information on a variety of topics, but may not have had an opportunity to apply this information in a "real world" setting.
2. Their experience has generally been limited to giving comprehensive care to two or three patients. If they have received team leading experience, it is usually limited in time and number of patients.

3. Their schedules have been almost entirely (in some cases entirely) limited to working during the day, Monday through Friday.
4. In most cases attendance has not been compulsory—a student can cut classes or even clinical experience with few repercussions.
5. Preparation for practice has consisted in large part of class discussions about nursing problems; these discussions tend to end with one correct answer to the problems.
6. Evaluation of students is given in a few clearly defined ways, always from instructors designated as having the right and responsibility to evaluate.

Some may say that the above characteristics do not hold true for the diploma graduates, but the nature of today's diploma programs must be taken into consideration. Various laws limit the number of hours per week students can spend in classroom and clinical work combined, so experience with patient care is not as extensive as it used to be. Since the student nurses can no longer be used to staff the units, the cost of hospital programs is becoming prohibitive. It is this fact, combined with the increasing emphasis on college degrees, that is sounding the death knell for diploma programs.

ADJUSTMENT TO HOSPITAL WORK

These characteristics of new graduate nurses cause adjustment problems when the newcomers enter the work world. Suddenly they are catapulted into an environment where they are expected to be on time, with required attendance, and care for large numbers of patients who present complex personal and physiological problems for which there are no "neat" answers. They are evaluated by everyone they come in contact with, from the person who sweeps the floor to the attending physician, and all too often they perceive these evaluations to be negative.

Brief et al. found that student nurses expect their role as practicing nurses to include professionally valued task demands such as patient instruction and counseling. When they discover that employing hospitals define the nurse's role as consisting largely of routine task demands, the differences encountered lead to role stress.[1] Another significant finding was that role stress is not improved by time on the job.[2] This means that the length of employment alone may not be enough to socialize new graduates to the work environment. Some sort of assistance must be built in to aid in the transition from student to employee.

Identifying Specific Problems

The first step in deciding what to offer for new graduate orientation is problem analysis. Each institution should design a questionnaire for nurses hired directly after graduation. The purpose is to discover their feelings about themselves, their preparation, and the problems they anticipate. Exhibit 10–1 shows a sample questionnaire. Such an open-ended form elicits general feelings and opinions that can provide valuable data for the orientation instructor.

Borovies and Newman reported that new graduates did not feel competent in performing a majority of clinical skills and felt unable to organize and delegate effectively.[3] In an extensive study of new graduates, procedures and experiences were ranked by the graduates as least and most difficult. Least difficult included changing dressings, giving medications, talking to patients, suctioning, and giving general patient care. Most difficult included working with physicians, doing catheterizations, recognizing and performing in emergencies, assuming charge nurse duties, and caring for dying patients.[4]

In a national survey conducted by Kramer and Schmalenberg, 196 recent graduates working in 13 large hospitals listed their top three goals as:

1. To test out my speed, ease, and competence in functioning as a staff nurse.
2. To see if I am competent in technical skills and procedures.
3. To try out my interpersonal skills in working with patients and families.[5]

In the same survey, 305 head nurses and supervisors working in the same hospitals as the graduates listed the goals they thought the new graduates should achieve. Their top three were:

1. Organizational skills and time management ability
2. Planning and giving care to large groups of patients
3. Developing speed, ease, and competence in functioning as a staff nurse.[6]

These differing priorities could be identified as yet another potential problem.

A study aimed at discovering what needed to be taught in a new graduate orientation program found that no areas of content can be eliminated from the orientation of any particular group of graduates. Not only were graduates of all three types of basic preparatory programs found to lack understanding of the nursing process for predicting and evaluating nursing care, but there was a wide range of skills and knowledge within the different baccalaureate programs alone. Evidence from this study suggests that it is not possible to predict content needed on the basis of educational program and that neither associate degree, diploma, or baccalaureate programs have identified the core content needed in the acute care setting.[7]

Exhibit 10–1 Sample New Graduate Questionnaire

New Graduate Nurse Orientation

1. What is your name? ______________________________
2. Where are you from? (school and area) ______________________________
____
3. Why did you choose nursing as a career? ______________________________
____
____
____
____
4. What, to you, is the scariest thing about this job? ______________________________
____
____
____
____
5. What do you think will be the best thing about this job? ______________________________
____
____
____
____
6. Do you feel that your nursing school did a good job preparing you for a nursing career?
____
____
____
7. Please share anything else about yourself that would help me to know you better. ______
____
____

Source: Education Department, Huntington Memorial Hospital, Pasadena, California. Reprinted with permission.

The implication for orientation instructors is clear: new graduates are not prepared to function as full-fledged staff nurses immediately after graduation. A traditional program designed to orient experienced nurses will not offer enough information, practice, or support for a newly graduated nurse. If your hospital hires new graduates, there are several questions that must be asked at the outset:

1. What sort of program or approach to new graduate orientation should be chosen?
2. What content should be offered, and how should it be sequenced?
3. How much time, money, and other resources is the hospital willing to devote to orienting new graduates?

LENGTH AND TYPE OF PROGRAM

Typically a new graduate program begins with general nursing orientation to which are added classes on pharmacology, team leading theory, care planning, communications, and the contributions of other departments to patient care. Many new graduates perceive such a program to be merely an extension of school, and if there is one thing they don't want more of, it's school. If they don't feel a need to learn something, it is very unlikely that the information will be retained.

Friesen and Conahan found that new nurses are action oriented, with much of their interest and energy absorbed in the new situation, relationships, and roles. If new graduates are offered classroom activities instead of the direct nurse-patient relationships they want and need, they often refer to such orientation classes as boring and irrelevant.[8]

When Schmalenberg and Kramer studied nurses in different types of new graduate programs, they found that comments on boredom were most common among new graduates in the most prolonged orientation programs.[9] In an attempt to ease new nurses into their roles, some institutions have set up orientations lasting many months. At some point, however, new graduates must be allowed to "try their wings." The very long programs may be overprotection, leading to frustration and boredom for the very people these hospitals are trying to help.

How long should a program be? There are no magic numbers. Different programs range from one week to over a year, and as yet no one approach can be proven to be the definitive one. What kind of program should be developed? There are four basic approaches to new graduate orientation: (1) extended orientation with special seminars, (2) use of preceptors, (3) internships, and (4) bicultural training.

Extended Orientation

Extended orientation programs are used most widely by hospitals, although more and more are trying the less traditional approaches as information regarding them is published in the literature. New graduate orientation programs generally provide all participants with similar experiences. After the standard nursing orientation, a new graduate spends more time on the units without being counted as staff and is usually given more time in class. Exhibit 10–2 is an example of an extended orientation for new graduates that is six weeks in length. After the first two weeks of regular orientation, participants work an additional month as orientees. Within that month they attend four seminars containing content considered important by the hospital. Rap sessions are also offered, where the graduates meet with a moderator to discuss problems.

Exhibit 10–2 New Graduate Orientation Schedule

New Graduate Program

Orientee __________ Head Nurse __________

Unit __________ Orientation Instructor __________

Monday	Tuesday	Wednesday	Thursday	Friday
8:00-4:30 New Employee Orientation	8:00-4:30 Nursing Orientation	8:00-4:30 Basic Cardiac Life Support	8:00-4:30 New Employee Orientation	7:00-3:30 UNIT (Buddy System)
8:00-4:30 Nursing Orientation	8:00-4:30 Nursing Orientation	7:00-3:30 UNIT (Work with Charge Nurse)	7:00-3:30 UNIT Total Patient Care	7:00-3:30 UNIT Total Patient Care
7:00-3:30 UNIT Total Patient Care	7:00-3:30 UNIT Total Patient Care	7:00-3:30 UNIT Total Patient Care	7:00-3:30 UNIT Total Patient Care	8:00-4:30 NEW GRADUATE SEMINAR
7:00-3:30 UNIT Buddy System with Team Leader	7:00-3:30 UNIT Buddy System with Team Leader	7:00-3:30 UNIT Team Leader for 6 Patients	7:00-3:30 UNIT Team Leader for 10 patients	8:00-4:30 NEW GRADUATE SEMINAR

7:00-3:30 UNIT Team Leader for 10 Patients	7:00-3:30 UNIT Full Team Leading	7:00-3:30 UNIT Full Team Leading	7:00-3:30 UNIT Full Team Leading	8:00-4:30 NEW GRADUATE SEMINAR
	Hours and assignments made by head nurse			NEW GRADUATE SEMINAR GRADUATION PARTY!

Source: Education Department, Huntington Memorial Hospital, Pasadena, California. Reprinted with permission.

Selection of Content

The areas of content that could be covered in a program for new graduates are almost limitless. Ask any group of nursing administrators—you'll get a long list of skills and knowledge that they feel are often lacking in new graduates, usually in the realm of organization and team leading. Ask a group of staff nurses and you will get another set of answers, probably dealing with teamwork, speed, and interpersonal skills with physicians and staff. And if you ask new graduates, the chances are you will receive quite a different set of answers, these dealing with nursing skills and procedures, patient-centered concerns about support and communication, and a deep desire to feel confident and competent in the new environment.

How can these differing viewpoints be reconciled? Perhaps a better question is: do they really need to be addressed in an orientation program? The first task of the orientation instructor may be to meet with nursing leadership and staff and discuss new graduates and what it is fair to expect from them. For instance, the best class in the world is not going to make a new graduate "organized." The ability to plan ahead and give care in an order and manner calculated to accomplish the most good in the least amount of time is developed only through experience. Some nurses never develop this ability, no matter how long they work—it certainly should not be expected of a neophyte.

As far as teamwork, speed, and ease of communication with physicians and staff are concerned, discuss with the other staff the fact that in school students work alone, with only their instructors for input and feedback. They are usually not encouraged to talk with the hospital staff to any great extent, for fear of "bothering" them or "getting in the way." If anyone doubts this, have them think back to the last time there were student nurses on the floor. It will take time for new nurses to consider themselves as part of the team, and only the staff can help them feel comfortable communicating with the different disciplines involved in patient care. As for speed, how realistic is that expectation for *any* nurse new to the environment and unfamiliar with layout, equipment location, forms, and the system of care delivery? New graduate or not, an orientee should be expected, even encouraged, to take enough time to thoroughly learn the methods and expectations of the unit before carrying a full patient load.

The expectations of the new graduates themselves are at once the most and least realistic. Certainly, the need to develop proficiency with basic nursing skills and procedures is deeply felt, and early orientation to the skills that will be used immediately is vital. Performing these techniques will help satisfy the new nurse's need to feel competent. The patient-centered concerns stem from graduates' perceptions of what constitutes good patient care, and is likely to be an area where they will be especially able. If the head nurses show that they value talking with patients and offering support, it will go far in making the new nurses accepted members of the unit team. Only time and support will achieve the third and most desired goal: to perceive themselves as competent nurses, to achieve a feeling of confidence in what they are doing.

After these initial meetings to clarify expectations and bring them closer to reality, objectives for the program are prepared, usually by the instructor with input from the line managers and staff. These objectives usually encompass only the orientation period, and are used in addition to the regular nursing orientation ones. Exhibit 10–3 is an example of such objectives. These focus on behavior changes related to content the new graduates receive in the classroom, hence the very specific actions required.

Using such a structured approach, how can the program be individualized to accommodate the needs of the participants? Unfortunately, if you are dealing with large groups of 30 or 40 graduates, it may prove impossible to individually tailor the program with any degree of success. One way to identify participant needs is through the use of a questionnaire given out in the first seminar. Exhibit 10–4 is an example of a form designed to elicit the expectations and needs of the graduates.

Once the questionnaires are completed, the information can be used to alter the program to meet stated needs. If the group is small, entire classes can be dropped or added. In a larger group, build in "cushions," where changes can be made without causing chaos. For instance, Exhibit 10–5 shows a content outline for a new graduate program containing five separate seminars. In the first seminar, topics are general, covering information needed by everyone. After that, data from the questionnaires can be used to alter content within the broad topic areas. For instance, equipment/procedure review in the second seminar should cover what the new graduates need. With one group the time could be spent demonstrating and practicing tracheal suctioning, tracheostomy care, major dressing changes, and use of the Clinitron bed. Another group might come up with an entirely different set of topics. If such things as injection techniques, piggyback IVs, and infusion pumps are not covered in regular orientation, they might be requested at this point. Porter found that the more directly the learning process relates to the problems experienced in the clinical situation, the more valuable to the graduates it will be.[10] The information planned for the seminars includes such immediately needed topics as care of ostomy patients, tips on organizing patient care, and interpreting laboratory values.

The presentation called "Life Management on the Night Shift" is given by a supervisor on the night shift who advises the nurses on how to cope with shift rotation and its impact on life style and health. No matter what shift graduates are hired on to, eventually almost everyone will work nights, and few have ever done so. Many of the tips work equally well for people going to the evening shift.

"Dissecting Roles in a Code Blue" addresses the intense anxiety new nurses have about functioning competently in emergency situations. The class begins by assessing the level of experience within the group (see Exhibit 10–6). Generally,

Exhibit 10–3 Objectives for New Graduates

New Graduate Orientation Program Objectives

Upon completion of the New Graduate Program, the orientee will be able to:

1. State which of her/his personal goals were met, and institute a plan for meeting other personal goals for the next six months.
2. Identify resources within H.M.H. available to help with professional, educational, and personal problems.
3. Confront her/his feelings about issues in nursing such as professional roles, nurse-physician relations, educational preparation, etc.
4. Perform most technical skills and procedures competently; and feel comfortable asking for help when encountering something unfamiliar.
5. Recognize the effect of her/his interactions on others and be able to use different approaches based on evaluation of others' responses.
6. List the phases of "Reality Shock" and identify some of the common reactions present in each phase.
7. Identify several self-tests and other tests on the clinical area and decide if the criteria used are valid and fair.
8. Elicit feedback from at least two persons on her/his clinical performance, and express agreement or disagreement with the feedback.
9. Function competently in a Code Blue situation as either the recorder, the "runner," or the nurse administering CPR.
10. Explain the system of organized patient education at H.M.H. as to: role of the Patient Education Specialist, resources available, Patient TV system, and the role of the unit nurse.
11. Given a set of patient situations, decide what actions you would take in what order and defend your decisions to the class group.
12. Identify the tasks and responsibilities of a team leader and lead a full patient team under the guidance of the charge nurse, nurse-clinician, or team leader.
13. Identify the equipment and resources available to care for a patient with an "ostomy" and for a patient with a decubitus ulcer.
14. List one advantage and one disadvantage for each of the four common styles of leadership; and discuss the role of leadership styles when group consensus is the objective.
15. Identify her/his dominant style of handling conflict and practice several different conflict strategies during simulated situations.
16. List the qualifications for an approved continuing education course and evaluate offered courses for quality, as well as stating the individual nurse's responsibility in meeting C.E. requirements for relicensure.
17. State the clinical significance of laboratory values for a variety of commonly ordered tests.

the graduates have not been involved in code situations; if they have seen one it has been strictly as an observer. Now they will be expected to work within the emergency response team as a full-fledged participant, with saving a patient's life as the outcome. The perception is terrifying. Discussion delineates who is respon-

Exhibit 10–4 New Graduate Questionnaire

1. What are your expectations relative to the new graduate position? ____________________

2. What are your goals for the next five weeks in relation to your nursing career? ____________________

3. What information and skills do you expect to receive from the new graduate seminars? ____________________

4. How do you feel about nursing *right now*? ____________________

Source: Education Department, Huntington Memorial Hospital, Pasadena, California. Reprinted with permission.

sible for what during a code procedure. Then the nurse's role specifically is dissected in detail. What must be done? When? How? What judgments must be made? A crash cart is opened. Where are drugs and equipment kept? How is the cart organized? What do frequently used pieces of equipment look like (a tonsil suction tip, for instance)? A videotape of a simulated cardiac arrest and the health team's response is shown, and the graduates must chart what happens on sample arrest record forms. After group members have had a chance to go through the cart (using the "Beat the Clock" game seen in Exhibit 4–4) and review the chart forms and responsibility sheets, mock codes are run with Resusci-Annie serving as the patient and the orientation instructor as the physician. Each participant has a chance to serve as a team member during a mock code. Those not directly participating observe the process and critique the team response.

The classes on Reality Shock do not so much present content (although Kramer and Schmalenberg's research is reviewed) as address the problems being encoun-

Exhibit 10–5 Outline of Seminar Content

I. First Seminar
   A. Introduction of facilitator and participants
   B. Review of program and objectives
   C. Explanation of orientees' roles in the program
   D. Break
   E. "How Do You See Nursing?"
   F. Lunch
   G. "Nursing Roles within the Patient Care System"
   H. Break
   I. "Styles of Communication"

II. Second Seminar
   A. "Life Management on the Night Shift"
   B. Break
   C. Equipment/Procedure Review
   D. Lunch
   E. "Reality Shock I"
   F. Break
   G. "Ostomy and Decubitus Care"

III. Third Seminar
   A. "Dissecting Roles in a Code Blue"
   B. Break
   C. "Getting Organized"
   D. Lunch
   E. "How To Lead a Nursing Team"
   F. Break
   G. "Styles of Leadership"

IV. Fourth Seminar
   A. "Reality Shock II"
   B. Break
   C. "Conflict Management"
   D. Lunch
   E. "Conflict Management," continued
   F. Break
   G. "Patient Teaching—How To Be an Expert"

V Fifth Seminar
   A. "Reality Shock III"
   B. Break
   C. "Everything You Always Wanted To Know About Pharmacology But Were Afraid To Ask"
   D. Lunch
   E. "Interpreting Laboratory Values"
   F. Wine and cheese party—and congratulations!

Exhibit 10–6 Code Blue Questionnaire

1. Have you ever participated as a team member in a cardiac arrest? ____________________
____
2. What is your biggest concern regarding your performance during an arrest situation? ____
____
3. How do you perceive the doctor's performance during an arrest? ____________________
____
4. How do you perceive your performance (real or imagined) during an arrest situation? ____
____
5. Do you feel you know what to expect (medications, procedures, responses, etc.) during this procedure? ____
6. Please state anything that might be done to help you prepare for a cardiac arrest situation:
____
____
____
____
____

Source: Education Department, Huntington Memorial Hospital, Pasadena, California. Reprinted with permission.

tered by the graduates and offer a nonthreatening environment for discussion and venting. If regular rap sessions are scheduled, this function happens there, also. The specific needs of the group can be met within the flexibility of this format.

What can you do if the new nurses express a major need that cannot be addressed within the structure of the seminars? For instance, suppose the pharmacology test results and the graduates themselves indicate that more information about drugs is desperately needed. Unless nursing administration wants to devote the time and money necessary to put the group through a pharmacology course, self-study is the only answer.

The graduates need guidance. Reading through their school pharmacology textbooks is not the answer. One way to help is to inform the group about what medications will be seen most often in the hospital, and then offer resources for self-study. Exhibit 10–7 shows a list of the medications most commonly encountered on the medical-surgical units of one hospital. Assist the new nurses in investigating the library; help them learn to use the nursing journals to extract current, patient-care-centered drug information. This approach establishes a habit of self-directed study within the nurses, so that they will continue to learn on their own throughout their professional careers.

Exhibit 10–7 Frequently Encountered Drugs

TYLENOL	AQUA-MEPHYTON	ATIVAN
CODEINE	BUTAZOLIDINE	PERITRATE
DIAMOX	ALDACTONE	COUMADIN
DYMELOR	RITALIN	CLINORIL
ELAVIL	HYOSCINE	REGLAN
ATROPINE $S0_4$	SERPASIL	HALDOL
URECHOLINE	PHENERGAN	VELOSEF
EDECRIN	VISTARIL	INDERAL
PREMARIN	MORPHINE $S0_4$	TORECAN
TENSILON	DEMEROL	PERCOCET
DOPAMINE	BANTHINE	TOLECTIN
VIBRAMYCIN	DONNATOL	PROBEC-T
LIDOCAINE	DILANTIN	NAPROSYN
PRONESTYL	TEGRETOL	MEBARAL
INDOCIN	TOBRAMYCIN	PERSANTINE
NALFON	SOMA	TRANSENE
DECADRON	ANCEF	LUFYLLIN
SOLUCORTEF	MOTRIN	LASIX
STREPTOMYCIN	SINEMET	ALUPENT
BENADRYL	GANTRISIN	ISORDIL
DIGOXIN	TIGAN	MINIPRESS
DARVON	CARBENICILLIN	FLAGYL
VALIUM	DIDRONEL	GENTAMYCIN
DIAZIDE	THEODUR	KEFLIN
ALDOMET	ZOMAX	INSULIN
ALDACTAZIDE	NITROL	QUINIDINE
HEPARIN	DILAUDID	TRIMETHOPRIM

Source: Education Department, Huntington Memorial Hospital, Pasadena, California. Reprinted with permission.

Unit Follow-up and Reinforcement

No matter what happens in the seminars, it is on the unit that new graduates put their knowledge and skills to work. How will they be accepted by nursing team members? Schmalenberg and Kramer discovered that new graduates stated that the treatment they received in the clinical area made them feel "nervous," "like dummies," or "incompetent to do the work."[11] Orientation instructors should meet with staff about the new graduate program, not only to clarify expectations, as mentioned before, but also to let them know content covered in orientation and how they can work effectively with their new colleagues. Check out whether the present staff remember their own orientation and can empathize with the newcomers. Unfortunately, although empathy is necessary for the staff to support and help orientees, research seems to indicate that nurses score lower on measures of empathy than most other occupational groups; indeed, one study reported that 71 percent of nurses showed *no evidence of empathy.*[12]

Having a clinician present in the unit who is responsible for orientation buffers new people during their adjustment period. Meisenhelder feels that the most important role of the unit teacher is helping the new graduate cope with the intense anxiety and fear of failing.[13] While some anxiety is helpful in learning, intense anxiety can inhibit the ability to assimilate and use new information. If the clinical instructor lowers this anxiety by explaining the values and expectations in the work setting to new people and by giving feedback on their behavior, orientees' self-esteem will be enhanced.

People with high levels of self-confidence and insight into their own coping mechanisms adjust to the demands and frustrations of nursing much more rapidly than those with less insight and lower self-esteem; indeed, the individual's level of self-confidence is more important to professional adjustment than clinical skills and past experience.[14] Strategies to help new people develop ego-strength and coping mechanisms must be created.

The head nurse and unit teacher should meet with each new graduate to review goals, philosophies, experiences, and values. Discuss unit expectations and discover the new nurse's expectations of the job. Let graduates know that a feeling of stress and overload is normal, and that exhaustion is a rational reaction to suddenly increased responsibility. A plan for professional development can be agreed on and the responsibility for it clearly placed on the new graduate. This is an important point. Although instructors and unit personnel can offer help and support, the final responsibility for making the adjustment can only belong to the individual. Orientees are being paid to attend seminars, learn needed information, put it into practice, and become functioning members of the health care team.

The strategies for clinical orientation discussed in Chapter 9 may apply to new graduates, but more time is required. Most new nurses need to know not only routines of care and how the hospital systems work but also how to make judgments and decisions necessary to being an excellent caregiver. One way to accomplish this is through participant observation, a strategy developed by Schmalenberg and Kramer. Newcomers observe a nurse chosen for the ability to make sound decisions, not working with a model, but observing the performance of patient care and asking the rationale for the actions taken and the decisions made.[15] This enables new graduates to discover the meanings that the models themselves give to their behavior. Use a number of experienced nurses, so that new people can observe different interpretations of like data and can learn the decision-making process itself rather than merely mimicking one nurse's actions.

Each new graduate will adjust to the system differently. One new nurse may be ready to lead a full team or work the night shift after a month's experience.

Another may not be ready for these high stress behaviors after two months have gone by. But this second nurse may blossom into an excellent team leader at the end of three months, after intensive patient care experiences, unit support, and self-study. If the system can also adjust to the new graduates and allow clinical expertise to develop slowly and thoroughly, the hospital, staff, graduates, and ultimately, the patients, will benefit.

USE OF PRECEPTORS

In a true preceptor-conducted new graduate program, there is no classroom component. Some experts are now recommending that the most effective type of orientation is to place the new graduates on the units where they will be working and then orient them immediately to the shift and role to which they will be permanently assigned.[16]

When this approach is used, the role of the clinical preceptor, as described in Chapter 9, becomes crucial. By introducing the new graduates to other members of the team and including them in both social and professional unit activities, preceptors support the newcomers' adjustment to their new roles. Unit preceptors also serve as role models, demonstrating the actions and judgment required of an excellent practitioner for the neophytes. In the unit-based programs, preceptors are responsible for all the teaching the new graduates receive.

In one successful preceptor program of this sort, the content taught each graduate is pertinent to the current activities of that nurse. While the overall information received by all new graduates is similar, timing is determined by the individual, and takes place in the clinical setting, not in a classroom.[17]

For this approach to work, preceptors have to be freed from their usual patient assignments in order to work closely with the graduates. It is not enough to let the orientees perform patient care under the supervision of the expert; the whole concept implies that the new nurses learn by watching an expert practitioner in action. Obviously, a mixture of observation, questioning, discussion, and teamwork is required.

The length of the precepting period must be totally individual, with the preceptor and the new graduate determining when and how the relationship will be gradually discontinued. Evaluation depends on the performance of the orientee, but the head nurse would meet with the preceptor at frequent intervals to obtain feedback on the orientation process and the new nurse's progress. In some hospitals the preceptors complete an assessment form on each new person they work with, and the form is used by the manager in evaluating the newcomer's progress. Some head nurses even include the preceptor in the evaluation conference, which could prove helpful if the preceptor is perceived as supportive by the orientee, but threatening if not.

Certainly, the orientees should have the opportunity to evaluate not only the program but the preceptors and their relationships with them. The only way such a program can prove beneficial is if the preceptors are selected with care (as described in Chapter 9), and if they support the new graduates through role transition in a way that protects and strengthens their all-important self-esteem and self-confidence.

INTERNSHIP PROGRAMS

Nursing internships developed by borrowing a concept from medical education and other disciplines. Intern programs are structured orientation programs that try to facilitate the transition from student to staff nurse through a prolonged period of supervised experience and classwork. One survey found that program length varied from six weeks to one year, with most programs running about 13 weeks.[18]

Internships might be considered work-study programs, in that the neophyte is essentially being paid to learn and is not considered a full staff member until the program is completed. Gibbons and Lewison found that 13 of the 14 intern programs surveyed paid the new graduates full salary throughout the whole orientation period.[19] In Roell's survey, only half the hospitals contacted paid full salary to nurse interns.[20]

When developing an internship program, administrative support is vital. Hiring a group of new graduates for an expensive and lengthy special orientation requires commitment of resources that could be used elsewhere. An internship program also requires a significant amount of direct supervision. Head nurses, clinical instructors or preceptors, and unit staff must be willing to guide the interns for a prolonged period while they cannot be counted as staff. Close, continual supervision appears to be a crucial element in all internship programs.[21]

If nursing administration is willing to wait for staffing vacancies to be filled when the interns complete the program, the orientation instructor generally coordinates the internship and provides the centralized classes that all participants attend. Content is chosen in the same way discussed in the section on extended orientation. In the intern programs surveyed, class content focused on technical skills, leadership techniques, and the application of problem-solving concepts to nursing problems, with the average time spent in class about 6.5 hours per week.[22]

Many programs rotate interns around the various units and shifts to thoroughly familiarize them with the hospital and to assist them in choosing a unit for permanent assignment. Coco surveyed intern programs to determine whether nurses adjusted to staff nursing and remained with the hospital after the program. Only 20 percent of the hospitals required a one-year commitment, but even though no contract was signed at most institutions, at least 50 percent of the interns did stay for at least a year.[23]

Respondents stated that their reasons for implementing such a program included:

1. Offer assistance with role transformation
2. Cope with new graduates' lack of experience and need for clinical skills
3. Eliminate duplication of teaching on the units
4. Improve quality of patient care
5. Serve as a recruitment tool.[24]

Internship programs may also help new graduates get a more realistic view of their skills and abilities, since the prolonged orientation period prevents an overwhelming onslaught of demands early in role adjustment. Rowland and Rowland found that many new graduates think they "can't do anything," and need several weeks to accurately assess their skill proficiencies as well as deficiencies.[25] Not being counted as staff through this crucial period may buffer the graduates enough to protect their self-esteem.

Roell reports that people closely associated with most intern programs report very positive results.[26] Besides subjective evaluations of the programs by the participants, retention rates are used as an objective measure of program effectiveness. In programs studied, the retention rates were cited as ranging from 50 to 100 percent, with an improvement in every institution.[27] There is no way to tell how much effect is obtained from the attention paid to the participants of these programs—a "Hawthorne Effect" (positive results due to the effects of the program itself rather than the content of the program or the changes made in the environment) could be at work, with retention rising because the new nurses feel cared for and nurtured. One expert warned that internship programs only "mitigate adjustment problems facing new graduates during the orientation period and to expect more is unrealistic."[28]

One rather striking finding was that associate degree nurses took approximately eight months to adjust to their roles while nurses from baccalaureate and diploma schools took four to five months.[29] This seems to imply that certain new graduates would derive more benefit from a longer program than others. Certainly, a hospital would want to examine its staffing needs, budget, and potential recruits before committing resources to such a comprehensive program. Careful assessment of the need for an internship program in your environment is a crucial first step that should not be skipped.

BICULTURAL TRAINING

Bicultural training is based on the research findings of Marlene Kramer and Claudia Schmalenberg. Studying large samples of newly graduated nurses, they identified a syndrome called Reality Shock, which they defined as "the shock-like reactions that occur when newcomers in an occupational field suddenly find that many of their professional ideals and values are not operational and go unrewarded in the work setting."[30] They found reality shock to be universal among new graduates, who adjust to the trauma in a number of ways, including job hopping, deserting their deeply felt ideals, or dropping out of the profession. In an effort to lessen the impact of reality shock, the two researchers studied this phenomenon in great detail.

Different phases of the experience were identified:

1. *Honeymoon Phase*—the initial reaction to actually working, having a paycheck, and being a "real" nurse is euphoria; everything about the situation is wonderful.
2. *Shock Phase*—a series of disillusioning events in which cherished values are shattered and denied precipitates the new graduate into a state of physical, mental, and emotional exhaustion and outrage in which the situation is perceived as being negative and hopeless.
3. *Recovery Phase*—eventually the shock victim regains a sense of perspective and the ability to laugh at the situation. Anger and tension reduce to manageable levels and creative problem solving can begin.
4. *Resolution*—although many new graduates resolve the conflict of leaving the situation, the most positive adjustment is a "bicultural adaptation" in which the new nurses meld their personal ideals to the ideals of the work place and function as both expert practitioners and creative managers of conflict and change.[31]

Bicultural training is designed to lessen the trauma of reality shock and hasten the development of biculturalism. Interpersonal competence is encouraged through the three components of the program:

1. *Affective*—a series of weekly seminars, approximately 90 minutes long, in which the graduates discuss what is happening in the work setting. These should take place in the shock phase, around six to eight weeks after they begin working.
2. *Cognitive*—the participants read and complete the modules contained in Kramer and Schmalenberg's *Path to Biculturalism.*
3. *Behavioral*—new graduates and their head nurses participate in several conflict resolution workshops which involve scripted role-playing. These are held four to five months post-hire.[32]

This approach is designed to provide new nurses with a support group of people undergoing the same experiences. Since all participants share the same values and all are at approximately the same level of experience, graduates can compare their performance and feelings to a fair standard, rather than to the more experienced nurses in unit work groups.

The orientation instructor serves as the group facilitator. Being in a staff position, the instructor is perceived as less threatening than a line manager and better able to preserve confidentiality. Special training in how to effectively conduct the seminars is strongly recommended; the facilitator role is difficult and delicate.

When Kramer and Schmalenberg compared bicultural training to traditional new graduate orientation, 260 new nurses employed in eight different medical centers were divided into two groups: a control group receiving traditional clinically based orientation and a study group receiving bicultural training. Both programs were matched in relation to time and format. Results demonstrated that the bicultural group had less turnover, instituted more changes in nursing practice, and received higher ratings from their supervisors.[33]

May, Minehan, and Deluty did a similar study in one institution only and found that while bicultural training increased interpersonal competence, tenure and performance were affected by multiple factors regardless of the type of orientation. As an example, the control group scored significantly higher on clinical knowledge and skills than did the bicultural group. The researchers investigated and found that the controls had attended more continuing education programs of a clinical nature, an indication that interpersonal competence is not a substitute for clinical competence.[34]

CHOOSING A PROGRAM

A review of the different programs discussed makes it clear that hospitals have a wide range of options available for orienting new graduates. The selection should be based on the individual institution's philosophy and available resources—and both these criteria must be in harmony. For instance, if your hospital offers a preceptor program for new graduates, provision must be made to train the preceptors *and* the staff so that they have time to support and instruct the new nurses. Costs are hidden within staffing patterns and may not be seen by the head nurses until the program is under way. At that point support for the program could suddenly be withdrawn and both preceptor and new graduate given a full patient assignment. This can be prevented by stating the costs during the planning stages and obtaining commitment from the managers involved *before* implementing the program.

In every case, these approaches to new graduate orientation are expensive. Internships usually cost the most, simply because of their length. Many hospitals absorb these costs as a recruitment strategy, but if your organization doesn't need to exert itself to recruit newly graduated nurses, that should be considered.

Some hospitals have found bicultural training to be less expensive than traditional new graduate programs.[35] Each situation is unique, so the experience of other institutions can be used only as a guide, not as a map. One approach might be to try several different programs on a pilot basis and compare results. Keep track of turnover, evaluations, and other measures of overall program effectiveness, and note how graduates completing the different approaches react to employment. Obviously, you will have no control over the subjects you get, so the samples cannot be matched, but your purpose is not rigorous research so much as simply getting a feel for which program will work best in your particular setting.

Ashkenas found that 78.8 percent of 313 new graduates studied identified their programs as helpful regardless of length. The few who saw orientation as a deterrent were in programs of less than a week in length or over six weeks, implying that duration of orientation may be a factor.[36] In the very long programs (such as internships) there could be a psychological component as well—do the participants tend to feel that they are being treated as students, not trusted with "adult" responsibility?

One important thing to keep in mind is the necessity of following through with implied promises to orientees. If new graduate orientation is described as a six-week program in which the participants will not be counted as staff and will receive individualized assistance, then that is what should happen. If confidentiality is guaranteed in seminars or rap sessions, the graduates should not later be approached by their head nurses for an explanation of why such-and-such was discussed in those sessions. If the hospital decides that new graduates will not receive any special orientation but will work directly on assigned units like any other nurse, that is a valid decision—as long as such a program is not described as an internship or some other deceptive term.

Since some studies seem to indicate that the process of job acclimation is fundamentally the same for new graduates as for experienced nurses, with adjustment to the organization the important process rather than role transition, emphasis on special programs for new graduates may be misplaced.[37] Weisman et al. feel that increasing efforts to orient and retain all staff nurses, regardless of experience, may prove to be a more practical approach to employment stability.[38] Whatever the approach chosen, orientation instructors will have a crucial role in developing and implementing the program.

CONCLUSION

New graduate orientation was developed in response to changes in nursing education. A variety of programs exist to prepare new nurses to adjust to full patient assignments and the decision making and problem solving that accompany the role of staff nurse. Decisions as to what type of program to develop rest on such criteria as cost factors, institutional philosophy and beliefs about orientation, and commitment of nursing managers to staffing patterns that support role transition and adjustment to the organization.

Chapter 11 will examine orientation to specialty areas. Once basic orientation is completed, nurses assigned to units such as critical care, obstetrics, pediatrics, surgery, etc., should receive instruction in the routines and equipment peculiar to those units. Programs covering this information will be described, along with the pitfalls that exist in implementing them.

NOTES

1. Arthur P. Brief et al., "Anticipatory Socialization and Role Stress Among Registered Nurses," *Journal of Health and Social Behavior* 20, no. 6 (June 1979): 162.
2. Ibid., 164.
3. Dianne L. Borovies and Nancy A. Newman, "Graduate Nurse Transition Program," *American Journal of Nursing* 81, no. 10 (October 1981): 1833.
4. Thais Levberg Ashkenas, *Aids and Deterrents to the Performance of Associate Degree Graduates in Nursing* (New York: National League for Nursing, Pub. No. 23–1465, 1973), 39.
5. Marlene Kramer and Claudia Schmalenberg, *Path to Biculturalism* (Wakefield, Mass.: Contemporary Publishing, 1977), 119.
6. Ibid., 120.
7. Deborah M. Schroeder, Marjorie M. Cantor, and Susan W. Kurth, "Learning Needs of the New Graduate Entering Hospital Nursing," *Nurse Educator* 6, no. 6 (November 1981): 16.
8. Laurel Friesen and Barbara J. Conahan, "A Clinical Preceptor Program: Strategy for New Graduate Orientation," *Journal of Nursing Administration* 10, no. 4 (April 1980): 18.
9. Claudia Schmalenberg and Marlene Kramer, *Coping with Reality Shock: The Voices of Experience* (Wakefield, Mass.: Nursing Resources, 1979), 79.
10. Sharon Ferrance Porter, "Interaction Modeling: An Educational Strategy for New Graduate Leadership Development," *Journal of Nursing Administration* 8, no. 4 (April 1978): 21.
11. Schmalenberg and Kramer, *Coping,* 98.
12. Marlene Kramer and Claudia Schmalenberg, "The First Job . . . A Proving Ground," *Journal of Nursing Administration* 7, no. 1 (January 1977): 14.
13. Janice Bell Meisenhelder, "The New Graduate Socialization," *The Journal of Continuing Education in Nursing* 12, no. 3 (1981): 21.
14. Ibid., 16.
15. Schmalenberg and Kramer, *Coping,* 148.
16. Ibid., 132.
17. Friesen and Conahan, "A Clinical Preceptor Program," 20.
18. Shelagh M. Roell, "Nurse Internship Programs: How They're Working," *Nurse Educator* 6, no. 6 (November-December 1981): 30.
19. Lillian K. Gibbons and Dana Lewison, "Nursing Internships: A Tri-State Survey and Model for Evaluation," *Journal of Nursing Administration* 10, no. 2 (February 1980): 32.
20. Roell, "Nurse Internship Programs," 30.
21. Gibbons and Lewison, "Nursing Internships," 32.

22. Roell, ''Nurse Internship Programs,'' 30.

23. Charlene D. Coco, ''A Report on Nurse Internship Programs,'' *Supervisor Nurse* 7, no. 12 (December 1976): 13.

24. Gibbons and Lewison, ''Nursing Internships,'' 34.

25. Howard S. Rowland and Beatrice L. Rowland, *Nursing Administration Handbook* (Rockville, Md.: Aspen Systems Corp., 1980), 236.

26. Roell, ''Nurse Internship Programs,'' 29.

27. Ibid., 30.

28. Ibid.

29. Coco, ''A Report on Nurse Internship Programs,'' 12–13.

30. Kramer and Schmalenberg, *Path to Biculturalism,* 4.

31. Ibid., 6–24.

32. Suzanne Diffey Holloran, Barbara Hyduk Mishkin, and Birdie L. Hanson, ''Bicultural Training for New Graduates,'' *Nurse Educator* 5, no. 1 (January-February 1980): 9.

33. Ibid., 8.

34. Louise May, Paula J. Minehan, and Linda Deluty, ''Evaluating Bicultural Training,'' *Journal of Nursing Administration* 11, no. 5 (May 1981): 29.

35. Holloran, Mishkin, and Hanson, ''Bicultural Training,'' 13.

36. Ashkenas, *Associate Degree Graduates,* 27.

37. Carol S. Weisman et al., ''Employment Patterns Among Newly Hired Hospital Nurses: Comparison of Nursing Graduates and Experienced Nurses,'' *Nursing Research* 30, no. 3 (May-June 1981): 191.

38. Ibid.

Chapter 11

Orientation to Specialty Areas

Besides requiring the orientation of all nurses, the Joint Commission on Accreditation of Hospitals mandates that nurses working in special care areas be given formal education relating to those areas.[1] Going into a specialized unit requires knowledge and skills not covered in basic nursing education programs. If nurses are brought into these areas without receiving additional instruction, they will be unable to make appropriate patient observations, handle the equipment properly, or give safe, effective care.

All orientations to specialty areas have the same goal: by the end of the special orientation, the theory level of the orientee should be close to that of the staff in that area. Note that no reference is made to the level of *practice*—it is hardly realistic to expect a person new to a specialty to perform at the same level of expertise as an experienced practitioner. But knowledge of the unique problems, equipment, situations, disease states, and nursing interventions should be provided before the nurse begins caring for patients.

Usually, nurses going to specialty areas participate in regular hospital orientation and then move into special classes relating to their specialty. Problems that must be addressed include:

1. Who will be admitted to the program? Will there be any educational or experiential requirements?
2. Should a qualifying examination be required?
3. What content should be presented before the end of orientation?
4. What sort of clinical reinforcement and follow-up should be provided?
5. How will the orientees—and the program—be evaluated?

REQUIREMENTS FOR ENTRY

Hospitals have varying philosophies about what experiences or knowledge should be required for entry into a specialty area. Some institutions will accept only nurses experienced in the area they are applying for, others will accept people new to the specialty if they have taken a course covering the theory involved (such as critical care classes). In both these instances, the responsibility for preparation rests on the nurse alone. Other hospitals offer courses as part of orientation that are designed to take nurses with basic education and prepare them to practice in a specialty.

The criteria for such a decision encompass two areas: recruitment and quality assurance. If your hospital has difficulty getting enough nurses to staff the special care areas, educating orientees may be the only answer. Some institutions have the philosophy that the only way to guarantee that all specialty staff practice at the level of expertise required is for all nurses entering a specialty area to participate in the hospital's own preparatory program. Therefore, they require all orientees, regardless of prior education or experience, to go through the specialty courses before beginning practice. Of course, costs should be considered when setting up such a policy—each nurse oriented to a specialty unit costs the hospital between $1,000 and $3,000 over and above the cost of regular orientation.[2] That figure could probably be considered conservative.

If tests are used to determine how much orientation is needed by each individual nurse, the examination must be validated before being used for evaluation purposes. The test should be given to a representative sampling of nurses currently working in the specialty and an item analysis done on the questions. Any questions missed by 40 percent or more of the subjects should be thrown out or revised. It is unfair—and subject to appeal at the Labor Board—to require orientees to pass a test that the current staff cannot pass.

Another decision that must be made is whether or not new graduates should be allowed to go directly to specialty areas from school. In the pressure to achieve full staffing and compete with other hospitals for new nurses, some hospitals send new graduates straight into specialties once basic hospital orientation is completed. Moyer and Mann found that neophytes had no chance to gain confidence in the new role of registered nurse when immediately confronted with the role of critical care nurse practitioner. Crying episodes and persistent thoughts of quitting during orientation were common. The process of becoming a competent practitioner was accomplished with greater ease when the new graduates had experience prior to employment in critical care.[3]

Houser did a study identifying predictors of performance levels in special care units. An analysis of educational background, previous clinical experience, and test scores revealed that previous clinical experience was a significant predictor of successful job performance, but only when related to the other two variables. High or very low test scores tended to be more predictive of performance than the middle range. The basic educational program was a significant predictor only for the associate degree graduates. Occurrence of low performance levels in 100 percent of the sample even after six months of employment was noted.[4]

The major finding of the study was that successful job performance in special care areas takes three months for an experienced nurse to achieve, as opposed to six months for one with no prior experience.[5] This supports the idea that practice in medical-surgical areas, becoming familiar with basic procedures and patient care management, is helpful before trying to master more complex care processes. The high occurrence of performance problems in the associate degree graduates could reflect limited clinical experience or it could be a sample problem. Since follow-up ended at six months post-hire, this group may just have taken longer to adjust to the special care environment.

PRESENTATION OF CONTENT

Content of the specialty programs should be selected just as content for general nursing orientation is chosen: line managers and staff decide what information is needed by new people to provide a firm foundation for safe, effective patient care. This will obviously vary from specialty to specialty and from hospital to hospital. Once the basic content is known, the educator plans how to cover it quickly and effectively.

In a survey of hospitals offering special care orientation, informal instruction (one-on-one discussion/demonstration of care) was designated as the primary method of presentation by 79 percent of the units. In addition, 91 percent of the units provided some formal instruction as well, and self-study was used by 86 percent.[6]

A hospital using a mixture of formal and informal instruction scheduled the classes for one day a week for six weeks to provide an opportunity for the orientees to get practical experience with special care patients and thus relate it to the theory being covered. Instructors in the program found that the nurses were able to participate more fully in classroom discussions, and greater exchange of information took place.[7]

Another orientation program used a programmed instruction approach to cover specialty information. This self-study method placed responsibility for learning content on the individual orientees, who covered the various modules at their own speed. Independent study was found to be as effective a method for special care orientation as traditional classroom instruction, and the orientees viewed it as more satisfying.[8]

Learning laboratories have also been used to demonstrate clinical skills to the orientees. Learning to operate special equipment and perform unfamiliar procedures is best done in a simulated setting. If practiced for the first time in the clinical area, patient and orientee anxiety are likely to be overwhelming and interfere with learning.

Content can be presented in a number of ways in specialty programs, depending on the resources and expertise of the instructor. Cost factors must also be considered. Large groups can be less expensively taught in a formal classroom setting; as the number of participants drops, costs rise. One-on-one instruction can be expensive because of the instructor time involved, but when combined with patient care—as in a preceptor program—cost effectiveness is easier to prove. Self-study modules are costly to develop and require training in techniques of programmed learning, but once prepared they can be used over and over again. And a learning laboratory for special care requires extremely expensive equipment and supplies, though the cost of setting one up may be defensible on the grounds of developing increased self-confidence and clinical proficiency in orientees.

CLINICAL REINFORCEMENT AND FOLLOW-UP

The experience gained in the clinical setting reinforces and strengthens knowledge covered in the theory component of orientation. Responsibility for the development of clinical skills is usually shared by the manager and a designated staff person (such as the preceptor). As in regular nursing orientation, clinical assignments are crucially important. If the new person is brought along too quickly, especially in the high stress environment of a specialty unit, dissatisfaction and ego threat will lead to a high turnover rate. Taking the cost of specialty orientations into consideration, hospitals cannot afford this cycle.

In the survey of specialty units, 91 percent of the units said they used a written orientation plan and 60 percent stated that orientees participated in planning their own orientations, either through self-assessment of needs and skills, selection of assignments, or goal setting and formulation of objectives.[9] Involving orientees in activities such as these not only follows adult education principles, but also may lessen the threat of a complex, lengthy orientation plan that seems overwhelming when first presented.

How long should specialty orientation last? In the surveyed institutions, 79 percent of the programs were between three and eight weeks in length, 18 percent were eleven to twelve weeks long, and three units had programs longer than 16 weeks.[10] Add to this the required general nursing orientation, and the shortest specialty orientation is six weeks in length. This means that managers and staff have a fairly limited amount of time to bring the orientees to an acceptable level of knowledge (theory) and expertise (practice).

During unit orientation in the specialties, one social phenomenon often occurs that the preceptor or other designated staff person should watch for and try to minimize. Nurses working in specialties often develop an aloofness from other staff based on the special knowledge and skills required in these areas. This perception of being "the elite" has benefits in developing camaraderie and partially compensating for the stress often involved in specialties. However, when new staff arrive, this very exclusiveness can cause problems for orientees. Humphries found that operating room nurses will be socially pleasant but professionally suspicious until the new nurse has proven to be hard-working and knowledgeable about all aspects of nursing *except* the operating room. In that area, they expect new nurses to recognize a deficit, and they are eager to give instructions and guidance.[11] A similar phenomenon is seen in most specialty areas, and the potential for problems with new graduates who are not yet able and confident in general nursing is obvious. Even less likely to be accepted is the experienced nurse who claims clinical expertise in the specialty and then is unable to perform to the standards of the other staff—social and professional ostracism will result.

A preceptor can buffer new staff from these chilling effects by working with them on patient assignments, rather than assigning them to their own patients. Observing expert care and modeling the preceptor's behavior, new staff can win acceptance more easily. Also the preceptor can bring experienced staff to a more realistic appraisal of new people by persuading them to withhold evaluation until orientees become more familiar with the work environment, and by acting as advocate.

EVALUATION OF SPECIALTY PROGRAMS

Program evaluation will be covered in detail in Chapter 14, but specialty orientation programs require a special emphasis on clinical evaluation. Since the bulk of these programs are conducted by unit personnel, follow-up and judgments about effectiveness should be done at the unit level. Besides analyzing subjective measures of satisfaction or dissatisfaction about the program, managers can compare levels of care and productivity before and after program completion. Personnel measures such as turnover, performance evaluations, and exit interviews provide the hospital with indices of the impact different approaches to orientation have on orientees.

At one institution, implementation of a specialty orientation resulted in a 50 percent decrease in turnover of licensed personnel; 23 months before the orientation program began 75 percent of newly hired people resigned, but during a comparable period following the establishment of an orientation program only 25 percent resigned. Analysis of data from exit interviews supported the conclusion that the turnover decrease was attributable to the orientation program.[12]

SPECIALTY ORIENTATION PROGRAMS

Critical Care

In 1971 there were 3,200 intensive care beds in the United States; by 1979 there were 62,000.[13] The 1983 edition of *Hospital Statistics* listed a total of 80,794 intensive care beds (of all types) nationwide.[14] The numbers of critically ill patients who can be helped by the care given in intensive care, coronary care, and other areas geared to operation of newly available equipment will undoubtedly continue to grow. As the number of units grows, the number of specially prepared critical care nurses must also grow.

Since few basic nursing programs provide extensive preparation in critical care, hospital orientation programs may be the first exposure a nurse has to this sort of practice. According to Sullivan and Breu, 83 percent of the hospitals that have intensive care units provide special orientation for their new staff. The decision to offer such a program seems to be governed by size. Only 46 percent of hospitals with fewer than 50 beds have a critical care program; the figure is 95 percent for hospitals with 500 beds or more.[15]

Of these available programs, most seem to offer a combination of skills orientation and theoretical review of systems to prepare the new critical care nurse. Those hospitals that accept only experienced practitioners need only present information specific to the institution, but few seem able to require that kind of experience. In most areas, there just aren't enough critical care nurses to go around.

Systems review should cover all body areas, with special emphasis on the pulmonary, cardiovascular, and nervous systems. Beginning with a review of anatomy and physiology, each system should be covered in enough detail that orientees have a firm foundation in the pathophysiology and nursing implications of common disease entities encountered in critical care. Exhibit 11–1 is an example of the objectives of one segment of such a course. Note that these end behaviors focus on the nursing applications of the theory covered.

The content of this particular course segment is shown in Exhibit 11–2, including not only the theory of different disorders of the respiratory system but also the assessment skills needed to discover problems and the techniques of treatment.

Exhibit 11–1 Excerpt from Critical Care Objectives

The participant will be able to:

1. Describe physiologic dead space.
2. List two causes of airway resistance.
3. Define compliance.
4. List two things that can alter diffusion.
5. State the advantages and disadvantages of MA_1 and PR_2 ventilators.
6. Describe the disadvantages of oral airways.
7. List two reasons for intubation.
8. Identify the blood gas abnormality indicating that the patient has developed hypoventilation.

Exhibit 11–2 Excerpt from Critical Care Class Outline

I. Anatomy and Physiology Review
  A. Anatomy of pulmonary system
  B. Physiology
    1. Ventilation (normal ventilatory patterns)
    2. Tidal volume
    3. Dead space
    4. Compliance
    5. Blood flow
    6. Diffusion

II. Pathology
  A. Hyper and hypoventilation
  B. Respiratory failure
  C. Chronic Obstructive Pulmonary Disease
  D. Chronic Restrictive Pulmonary Disease

III. Physical Assessment
  A. Inspection
  B. Palpation
  C. Percussion
  D. Auscultation

IV. Treatments and Nursing Care
  A. Oxygen
  B. Humidification and nebulization
  C. Drugs (antibiotics, antispasmodics, bronchodilators, mucolytics)
  D. Airways (oral, nasal, E.T. tubes, tracheotomy)
  E. Mechanical ventilation

Thorough grounding in critical care theory and practice takes time. In the program discussed, covering all the systems would take six weeks, with a full day of class once a week. Clinical experience related to class content takes up the rest of each week. This time must be added after initial nursing orientation, so the total orientation time for a critical care nurse would be nine weeks. Nurses with no critical care experience would require more time, since they must have a two-week course in basic arrhythmia interpretation and a two-day certification in intravenous techniques.

The costs of such a program can rapidly become prohibitive, especially when individuals or very small groups are being oriented. Some hospitals are trying self-study as a way around this problem. In one such program, the entire content is taught in self-instructional units proceeding in small sequential steps with immediate feedback provided. The curriculum includes:

Cardiovascular Anatomy
Blood Pressure Physiology
Electrical Safety
Pacemakers
Anticoagulants
ECG Interpretation
Respiratory System
Arterial Blood Gases
Bird Respirator
Bennett Respirator
Chest Tubes
Fluids and Electrolytes
Shock
Congestive Heart Failure

Each of these topics is a self-contained study module.[16]

The choice of how to conduct critical care orientation must be made on the basis of the following factors:

1. Type of patients—how complex is the care and knowledge expected of the nurses?
2. Type of unit—what sort of equipment is available?
3. Orientees—how prepared are they for critical care?
4. Resources—who is available to cover the content? If no instructor with critical care experience is employed, unit personnel must carry the teaching burden.
5. Expectations—what level of knowledge and expertise is expected of these nurses when they complete the program?

Whether critical care orientation is presented in the classroom, via self-study modules, or through a combination of both methods, careful evaluation is necessary to determine each nurse's level of practice. Exhibit 11–3 is an excerpt from a test on the didactic material covered in the Pulmonary System class presented in previous exhibits. Another form of written examination calls for decision making by the nurse based on the problem presented (see Exhibit 11–4). This sort of test may measure application of theory more accurately.

The most reliable test of clinical knowledge and expertise is observation in the clinical area. Only by actually watching orientees deliver care can the managers or preceptors assure themselves that theory has been assimilated into practice. Observing orientees, reading their charting, keeping track of quality assurance measures—all these should be done systematically any time new people are oriented.

Operating Room

The OR specialty requires total preparation for any nurse who has not worked in surgery before, since most basic nursing programs no longer include operating room experience in the curriculum. Most orientees will not be familiar with the equipment, procedures, and routines of the area. Initial orientation periods range

Exhibit 11–3 Excerpt from Critical Care Examination

Respiratory System

1. Briefly describe compliance. ________________

2. Describe physiologic dead space. ________________

3. The blood gas abnormality indicating hypoventilation is ________________
4. List two causes of airway resistance.
   a. ________________
   b. ________________
5. List two factors that can alter diffusion.
   a. ________________
   b. ________________
6. List two indications for intubation.
   a. ________________
   b. ________________
7. State one advantage of an MA_1 ventilator over a PR_2.
   ____
8. List two disadvantages of oral airways.
   a. ________________
   b. ________________

from six weeks to six months, depending on the hospital.[17] For new graduates complete orientation to the operating room might take from 18 months to two years.[18]

Some programs will not accept new graduates, requiring at least a year of general nursing experience as a prerequisite. The objectives of such a program are shown in Exhibit 11–5. These overall objectives describe the role of the nurse in the setting; each segment of information would then have its own set of specific objectives (see Exhibit 11–6). A combination of classwork and supervised clinical experience is used to cover the content areas.

The specialized nature of the work in surgery makes close clinical supervision essential. Many programs assign every new nurse to a preceptor for the entire length of the program. These two nurses work together through the different special areas of surgery (general, orthopedic, neurological, etc.), with the experienced mentor sharing knowledge and decision making with the orientee. Groah feels that every effort should be made to permit new employees to function as surgical nurses as quickly as possible.[19] Maintaining long "student" status is frustrating and potentially demeaning to orientees.

Exhibit 11–4 Excerpt from Critical Care Test

Standards of Nursing Practice
for Critical Care

1. You have just taken over the care of a patient with a Swan-Ganz catheter and the PA waveform is unacceptably damped. List five reasons for inaccurate pressure transmission from the catheter tip to the transducer which could produce a damped waveform.

____

____

____

2. Describe the clinical significance of each of the following pressure measurements:
   a. Pulmonary Artery Systolic Pressure ______________________________

   ____

   b. Pulmonary Artery Diastolic Pressure ______________________________

   ____

   c. PCWP ______________________________

   ____

3. Under what circumstances are pulmonary artery diastolic pressures significantly different from PCWP values? In what way do they differ?

____

____

4. Describe the criteria used to judge acceptable vs. unacceptable waveforms in each of the following monitoring positions:
   a. Right atrial waveform ______________________________
   b. Pulmonary artery waveform ______________________________
   c. PCWP waveform ______________________________

Source: Karen Flynn, Critical Care Clinical Specialist, Huntington Memorial Hospital, Pasadena, California. Reprinted with permission.

Among the tools that can be used as resources for new nurses are procedure books, setup cards for each procedure, pictures of the various instruments either in notebooks or a card file, handouts from class, catalogs, and actual textbooks on surgery available on the unit. These materials can be studied when time allows and can also provide answers for employees when an instructor is not available.

Mackerty feels that new nurses should first scrub, then circulate in each service in order to keep procedures familiar and practiced.[20] This also follows the principle of moving from the simple to the complex as orientees learn routines and problems from the relatively "safe" position of scrub nurse before having to assume circulating nurse responsibilities. It is also recommended that new nurses spend time with the head nurse, unit secretary, and scheduling clerk to learn administrative and ancillary duties that may be needed on weekends and during charge experience.[21] Shift rotation, weekend duty, and call duty complete clinical experience as orientees gain confidence in their new roles.

Exhibit 11–5 Surgical Orientation Program

Course Description

This is a 9-month education program designed for the RN who has a minimum of one year general nursing experience and a sincere desire to increase his/her nursing knowledge.

Through the process of classroom instruction, workshops, and clinical rotations, the nurse will acquire the skills and proficiency of basic OR Nursing.

General Objectives

At the conclusion of the program the participant:

1. will understand that OR Nursing encompasses basic OR nursing practices plus specialty practices by incorporating and demonstrating these principles through the daily assignments.
2. after working with a mentor, will qualify to work independently and efficiently in the OR as a scrub nurse or circulating nurse in the less complicated specialties of surgery.
3. will be aware of, and practice on a daily basis, safety precautions in surgery in regard to self, fellow workers and patients.
4. through return demonstrations and daily practice, function as a role model and teacher of aseptic technique.
5. will be able to properly use, operate and care for surgical instruments, power equipment and special equipment relative to all specialties.
6. by participating in all types of surgery, will know the routine specifics for those types of surgery.
7. will demonstrate the ability to adequately and effectively assess the surgical patients' needs.
8. by means of assigned rotations will be able to function with minimal assistance in all areas of responsibility in the OR—i.e., scrub nurse, circulating nurse, charge nurse.
9. will display through daily assignments the ability to be a learner and a teacher.

This course is approved by the California BRN, Provider *#00351* for 30 contact hours.

Certificate will be issued at program completion.

Licensee must retain Certificate for a period of four (4) years following course completion.

Source: Surgery Department, Huntington Memorial Hospital, Pasadena, California. Reprinted with permission.

Testing and evaluation should be ongoing in a program as complex and detailed as operating room orientation. Besides traditional written tests, examinations can be prepared that evaluate ability to complete records properly and make appropriate nursing judgments. Exhibit 11–7 shows excerpts from a test requiring orientees to analyze forms, identify and correct errors, and completely fill out requisitions and other nursing records. Follow-up on this type of test can be done in the clinical area by examining the documentation completed by each nurse. Although

Exhibit 11–6 Specific Class Objectives

Concepts of Sterilization

OBJECTIVES

At the conclusion of the class, the participant will:

1. State:
   A. The four different types of sterilizers
   B. The necessity of having different types
   C. Modes of operation
   D. Advantages of each
   E. When to utilize one type as opposed to others
2. Through demonstration and practice sessions, be able to safely and independently, with 100 per cent accuracy, operate the three types of sterilizers located within the HMH surgery department.
3. Correctly package all types of items, using the proper packaging material and technique as identified through lecture and reading assignment.
4. Be able to define shelf life and apply the concept to her/his daily work by:
   A. Checking and rotating stock
   B. Pulling setups
   C. Opening a room
5. Perform on a routine basis all safety precautions of the decontamination process as identified through lecture and state the importance and necessity for decontamination.
6. State the correct guidelines for storage of supplies.
7. List the four required notations for the sterilizer record and write an explanation of this record's rationale.

Source: Surgery Department, Huntington Memorial Hospital, Pasadena, California. Reprinted with permission.

orientees may progress at slightly different rates, the end performance should meet agreed-on standards and objectives stated at the beginning of the course.

Obstetrics

Years ago obstetrics was considered a slow-moving, "easy" specialty where little additional theory was necessary. Except for the high pressure labor and delivery area, obstetrics required only the ability to hold babies, teach mothers, and soothe harried fathers. Today nurses in this specialty would laugh at that description. Advanced theories and procedures of perinatal and postnatal care enable them to save high-risk mothers and babies who would not have had a chance a few years ago.

The advent of high technology has converted postpartum and newborn nursery into areas delivering sophisticated nursing care—and labor and delivery into a

Exhibit 11–7 Excerpt from OR Nursing Records Exam

OR Nursing Records Exam

Page 1 represents a completed OR nursing record.

Indicate errors, deletions, etc., by a circle on the record in the particular location. On the answer sheet state:

1. What the error is, *and*
2. The policy or reason it is incorrect

If the line is correct, indicate by writing CORRECT on the answer sheet.

Page 4—According to the Nursing Record you completed, fill out the OR charge sheet for this case.

Page 5—According to the Nursing Record, complete the specimen slip and specimen tags.

Page 6—This chart coincides with the graph on page 7; mark the runs on this chart.

Page 7—This record represents four times that the sterilizer was turned on. You are the nurse who turned the sterilizer *off* each time. How would you mark the record?

Page 8—Complete this record (the specimen is a swab of the opened gallbladder).

1. Is there a time limit in which the specimen must go to the lab? YES NO
2. If the answer is yes, what is the time limit?

____

Page 9—Complete this record:

1. What is the surgeon looking for with this type of test?

____

____

2. Complete this blood request for one unit of whole blood. How many units can be ordered on this requisition?

____

Source: Surgery Department, Huntington Memorial Hospital, Pasadena, California. Reprinted with permission.

critical care area. Orientees must receive the theory and practice they need before venturing into situations requiring quick reactions and decision making. Most obstetrics areas assign orientees to postpartum first, both because their patient assignments can be better controlled and because this unit provides an overall view of the activities of the entire area. The care is more like that of a general nursing floor, which helps orientees make the transition easily. Classes cover care of normal and high-risk mothers from conception through and after delivery, since postpartum units often have a number of undelivered patients. Teaching skills are stressed, as patient instruction is an important duty in this area. Checklists and procedure books (see Exhibit 11–8) are valuable adjuncts to learning the routines of the floor.

Newborn nursery also provides special care and requires in-depth knowledge of both the normal newborn and the infant with problems. Assessment skills must be developed and practiced, since problems often signal their presence with almost indetectable signs that must be recognized and reported by the nurses. Classes cover the infant from birth to one month, stressing the role of the nurse in discovering and preventing problems, as well as the physical care of the normal newborn. Exhibit 11–9 is an example of objectives for a class preparing orientees to work in newborn nursery.

Labor and delivery requires nurses who can handle a great deal of pressure without the comfort of a set routine. Even intensive care and coronary care units generally have care routines—set times when medications and treatments are given, meal times for conscious patients, etc. In labor and delivery routine is almost nonexistent. Patients appear with little or no warning requiring instant

Exhibit 11–8 Excerpt from Maternity Procedure Book

11–7 Nurse Responsibilities

1. Takes report from 3–11 shift.
2. Checks NA assignment.
3. Checks Kardex against medication book.
4. Makes rounds on all patients immediately and every 30 minutes.
5. Administers medications as ordered.
6. Takes VS on patients as ordered.
7. Changes dates on addressograph at midnight.
8. Stamps new date on all charts (nurses' notes).
9. Checks Labor and Delivery census and prepares for admissions.
10. Files laboratory reports on all charts.
11. Goes through Kardex and completes laboratory slips for all ordered blood work. Tube to Laboratory.
12. Checks NA assignments and cleaning duties.
13. Reports to 11–7 supervisor at 4:00 A.M. rounds.
    Completes Unit Report and turns it in at that time.
14. Assists breast-feeding mothers as necessary.
15. Prepares any patients scheduled for surgery as ordered.
16. Charts on all patients.
17. Gives report at 7:00 A.M.

Exhibit 11–9 Excerpt from Nursery Orientation Objectives

The nurse will be able to:

1. list the Apgar categories and describe the criteria used to assign scores.
2. differentiate between primary and secondary apnea.
3. using a manikin, demonstrate correct CPR technique for a neonate.
4. using a manikin, demonstrate the correct way to operate ventilatory support equipment (such as Ambu bag) for a neonate.
5. list four ways heat loss can occur in the neonate and describe how to prevent each type.
6. draw and label the vessels in the umbilical cord.
7. describe acrocyanosis, mongolian spots, and milia. Explain how you would answer a mother's questions about each of these.
8. differentiate between caput succedaneum and cephalohematoma and describe the nursing implications of each.

delivery, or hemorrhaging, or needing an emergency caesarean section—which the nurse must arrange, set up, and then scrub for or serve as circulating nurse during the surgery. Some orientees find they simply cannot handle such an area. Individual hospital policy dictates whether they will be allowed to work postpartum or nursery or whether all obstetric nurses must be prepared to cover all three areas.

Obviously, labor and delivery should be the last area that nurses are exposed to during orientation. By the time they reach it they should have a firm foundation of knowledge and experience in the other two units, as well as classroom preparation for labor and delivery itself. The excerpt from an experience checklist in Exhibit 11–10 shows just a few of the skills required by orientees. In this area it is especially crucial that new nurses work with a preceptor of some kind. To simply turn an orientee loose without close guidance and supervision is not only unkind but actually dangerous.

The orientation to obstetrics is likely to be an extended one, sometimes taking six months for a new graduate to complete. Three months is probably the absolute minimum, allowing one month for each unit. Managers and educators use testing, observation, and other already described evaluation strategies to ensure that orientees can safely practice in all three units before releasing them to full staff status.

Pediatrics

Pediatric orientation varies greatly from institution to institution, depending on patient population. Some hospitals have small units basically concerned with

Exhibit 11–10 Excerpt from Labor and Delivery Checklist

Procedure	*Observed*	*Demonstrated*	*Notes*
Admission			
Fetal Monitoring			
External			
Internal			
Amniocentesis			
Induction			
Syntocinon			
Pitocin			
Vaginal Delivery			
Setup			
Notification			
Preparation of patient			
Nursing care			
Care of infant			
Post-delivery care			
Caesarean section			
Setup			
Notification			
Preparation of patient			
Scrub duties			
Circulating duties			
Care of infant			
Post-operative care			

minor surgery and an occasional trauma victim. Others have large, sophisticated units dealing with a wide variety of pediatric clients. In the first instance orientation might consist of little more than a review of child development, commonly encountered disorders, and special pediatric procedures, laboratory values, and equipment. In the second, detailed classes on a whole array of disorders and their accompanying assessment and treatment would be added to the curriculum. In either case, special emphasis must be given to dosage calculations and drug reactions for younger patients.

One area of pediatrics that is rapidly becoming its own specialty is the Neonatal Intensive Care Unit (NICU). Caring for premature and critically ill infants requires the use of complex instrumentation and constant assessment and response to life-threatening changes. The theory needed for such care includes a wide range of topics (see Exhibit 11–11). Spreading class days out enables orientees to meld observation and practice with theory into a coherent whole.

Exhibit 11–11 Outline of NICU Orientation Classes

1. Identification of high-risk pregnancy
2. Physiologic adaptations during transition
3. Fetal circulation
4. Thermoregulation
5. Physical assessment of the neonate
6. Cardiologic disorders
7. Hematologic disorders
8. Metabolic disorders
9. Care of the infant with respiratory distress
10. Neonatal drug administration
11. Surgical emergencies
12. Umbilical artery and vein catheterization
13. Neonatal cardiac, respiratory, and blood pressure monitoring
14. Neonatal infections
15. Neonatal nutrition
16. Infant transport
17. CPR
18. Nurse-parent communication
19. Grief and grieving
20. Discharge planning

Martin and Burnett recommend the use of a skills laboratory for NICU orientation. Such a laboratory simulates the patient environment by providing not only an isolette but also a radiant warmer, ventilator, vital signs monitor, resuscitation doll, intravenous pumps, pleurevacs, bag/mask/suction equipment, emergency medications, and intraflow/transducers. Skills can be demonstrated in this laboratory setting and return demonstrations performed without the stress of having actual patients present.[22]

Clinical practice requires one-on-one coaching and supervision to lower orientee anxiety and protect patients. The length of the program varies depending on the level of patient care delivered, preparation of the orientees, and institutional philosophy about orientation. Three months seems a reasonable length of time for formal orientation, although orientees might not be considered full staff members for up to six months, particularly if new graduates are admitted with no prerequisite experience.

Emergency Department

Similar to intensive care, emergency orientation requires special information and experiences to prepare new nurses for practice. Some programs use a combination of classes and clinical experience; others present the entire orientation on a one-to-one basis. Often the programs not offering classroom preparation require previous emergency experience. Exhibits 11–12, 11–13, and 11–14 show excerpts from a program conducted entirely in the clinical area.

The buddy system enables orientees to gradually assimilate information about the area and the delivery of nursing care. With close contact and daily conferences, preceptors obtain an accurate picture of the orientees' abilities and accomplishment of program objectives. Further development is encouraged through continuing education requirements, such as MICN certification.

Other Programs

Any area can use the specialty unit approach to orienting new employees. Any block of information required for effective practice can be transmitted to orientees through classroom work, self-study, one-on-one instruction, or clinical experience. For instance, Exhibit 11–15 shows part of an orientation checklist for an orthopedic unit in which theory and practice specific to the area is covered individually for each orientee, in addition to the information presented in regular nursing orientation.

Exhibit 11–12 Emergency Department Orientation

Purpose: This orientation program is to provide an introduction to the Emergency Department.

Objectives:
1. Have a working knowledge of the Emergency Department's purpose and organization.
2. Be familiar with his/her job description and the specific duties required.
3. Be familiar with the standards of care expected in the Emergency Room. Be able to function safely with some degree of autonomy in the primary care of emergency patients.
4. Be able to carry out Emergency Department policies and procedures.
5. Be familiar with the physical layout of the department and the location of equipment and supplies.
6. Understand the relationship our area has with other ancillary departments, such as radiology, lab, EKG, etc.

Name: ____________________________

Signature Upon Completion: ____________________________

Supervisor's Signature: ____________________________

A copy of the orientation manual will be kept in your personnel file.

Source: Emergency Department, Huntington Memorial Hospital, Pasadena, California. Reprinted with permission.

Exhibit 11–13 ED Orientation, Day One

Date		*Completed*	*Nurse Initials*
	1. Introduction to Huntington Memorial Hospital ED (organization/goals). 2. General introduction to staff (doctors, nursing, clerical, patient services, technicians). General introduction to the schedule, bulletin boards, lockers, lunch and break times, illness procedure, basic dress codes, clock-in, policy and procedure manual. Tour of physical layout of the ED. 3. Introduction to the nursing desk, charts (basic blank form), census, answering telephone. Sit with the cashier at the check-in desk for one hour. a. What information is asked and what is required? b. Follow the steps of making a chart. c. Note appropriate triage of patients. d. Note consents required. 1. General 2. Arbitration agreements 3. Emancipated minors 4. Witnessing of consents 5. Telephone consents 6. Emergency consents 7. Consent manual e. Presenting statements. f. Reportable cases—assault, dog bites, traffic collision. g. Incident reports. 4. Tour of Dispensary, PT, CSS, Maintenance, STAT Lab, and other departments on this floor. 5. Observation of department buddy while she/he is working. 6. Introduction to P.M. staff. Review of day and general overview of the second day's activities.		

Source: Emergency Department, Huntington Memorial Hospital, Pasadena, California. Reprinted with permission.

Exhibit 11–14 ED Orientation, Day Two

Date		*Completed*	*Nurse Initials*
	1. Review of first day's experience. 2. Orientation to Room 1 and Room 2 with buddy. a. Learn location of linen, oxygen, suction, and location of materials to resupply them. b. Learn how to operate each bed. c. Learn the location of the scale and how it operates. d. Learn the location of the ophthalmoscopes and their care and use. e. Acquaint yourself with what is in each drawer and cupboard, and where supplies are to resupply each article. f. Acquaint yourself with location and use of the call lights and side rails. g. Acquaint yourself with the types of patients most frequently admitted to these rooms. h. Learn how to operate each piece of equipment found in these rooms (IVAC, portable light, armboard, lavage equipment, tubex). i. Acquaint yourself with the equipment found in the cupboard outside Room 1. j. Review procedure for cleansing of wounds, suturing, and the application of dressings. 3. Buddy with nurse—observe and assist with patient care in rooms 1 and 2. 4. Review of the day and general overview of next day's activities.		

Source: Emergency Department, Huntington Memorial Hospital, Pasadena, California. Reprinted with permission.

Such an organized approach enables any unit to orient new nurses in a systematic way. Each person receives the same information in the same way rather than learning about the equipment, procedures, and routine in piecemeal fashion as each situation is encountered.

Exhibit 11–15 Orthopedic Orientation Checklist

Skill	*Knowledge Required*
Set up Buck's traction	Equipment/Procedure
Care of patient in skeletal traction Assessment Circulatory checks Bedmaking Pin care Exercises Teaching	Equipment/Principles/Physical assessment skills/Pathophysiology/Psychosocial assessment and interventions
Care of patient with hip fracture Positioning and turning Ambulation Skin Care Nutrition Teaching	Pathophysiology/Bone healing/Fracture care/Principles of ambulation/Nutrition/ Psychosocial assessment and interventions
Care of patient in cast Assessment Circulatory checks Skin care Cast care Crutch-walking	Physical assessment/Bone healing/Cast care/Skin care/Crutch-walking

CONCLUSION

Orientation to specialty areas involves a combination of classroom theory, self-study, and clinical experience. Programs range from three weeks to 18 months in length, with the majority between six and eight weeks long. The requirements vary with the level of care required in the unit and the previous experience of the orientees. If new graduates are admitted, extra time must be allowed for them to obtain the clinical expertise and confidence needed to function in these areas.

Chapter 12 covers orientation of people assisting nurses in delivering patient care: nurse attendants, orderlies, and unit secretaries. Without these adjunct personnel most units would cease to function, yet sometimes little thought or planning seems to go into preparing them for their vital roles. In the next chapter the pros and cons of training people from scratch as opposed to orienting only experienced people will be discussed and various programs will be presented.

NOTES

1. *Accreditation Manual for Hospitals, 1983 Edition* (Chicago: Joint Commission on Accreditation of Hospitals, 1983), 183.

2. Heidi Nerwin Hansell and Sue B. Foster, "Critical Care Nursing Orientation: A Comparison of Teaching Methods," *Heart and Lung* 9, no. 6 (November-December 1980): 1066.

3. Marilyn G. Moyer and James K. Mann, "A Preceptor Program of Orientation Within the Critical Care Unit," *Heart and Lung* 8, no. 3 (May-June 1979): 533–534.

4. Doris M. Houser, "A Study of Nurses New to Special Care Units," *Supervisor Nurse* 8, no. 7 (July 1977): 21.

5. Ibid., 22.

6. S. Manning, "Characteristics of Burn Orientation Programs," *Journal of Burn Care Review* 4, no. 1 (January-February): 50–51.

7. Martha D. Rieman, "Educational Approaches to Burn Nursing Orientation," *Journal of Burn Care Review* 4, no. 1 (January-February 1983): 31.

8. Hansell and Foster, "Critical Care Nursing Orientation," 1072.

9. Manning, "Burn Orientation Programs," 50.

10. Ibid.

11. Shirley Humphries, "Nurturing the Nurse: OR Orientation," *AORN Journal* 30, no. 1 (July 1979): 65.

12. Temme L. Martin and Patricia A. Burnett, "Development of a Neonatal Intensive Care Orientation Program," *Journal of Obstetric, Gynecologic, and Neonatal Nursing* 11, no. 3 (May/June 1982): 179.

13. Margaret D. Sovie, "Fostering Professional Nursing Careers in Hospitals: The Role of Staff Development, Part 1," *Nurse Educator* 7, no. 6 (Winter 1982): 31.

14. ________ *Hospital Statistics*, 1983 Edition (Chicago: American Hospital Association, 1983), 207.

15. Sadra Sullivan and Christine Breu, "Survey of Critical Care Nursing Practice, Part IV: Staffing and Training of Intensive Care Unit Personnel," *Heart and Lung* 11, no. 3 (May-June 1982): 239.

16. Martha C. Schmidt, "A Self-Paced ICU Core Curriculum," *Cross-Reference* 7, no. 2 (March-April 1977): 4.

17. Humphries, "Nurturing the Nurse," 64; Jacqueline Joseph Birmingham, "Clinical Orientation by Objectives," *Today's OR Nurse* 2, no. 7 (September 1980): 7.

18. Humphries, "Nurturing the Nurse," 64.

19. Linda Groah, "Staff Development—Reality Oriented," *AORN Journal* 24, no. 6 (December 1976): 1065.

20. Carolyn Kramer Mackerty, "Orientation Program for the New OR Nurse," *AORN Journal* 17, no. 5 (May 1973): 89.

21. Ibid., 90.

22. Martin and Burnett, "Neonatal Care," 177.

Chapter 12

Orientation of Auxiliary Personnel

Webster's Third New International Dictionary defines *auxiliary* as "offering or providing help, assistance, or support especially by interaction."[1] What better description could there be of the auxiliary personnel who provide so much care to our patients: nurse attendants (NAs), orderlies, and unit secretaries. Ever since the nursing shortage brought about by World War II, numbers of auxiliary personnel have grown amazingly. The overwhelming majority of hospitals in the United States use auxiliary workers as "nurse-extenders," where the nonprofessionals perform the less complex tasks in order to free nurses for patient care and assessment requiring professional judgment.

Since these workers have no professional preparation, careful orientation is vital. Whether you will be teaching a group of laypeople the entire job from the ground up or orienting experienced personnel to hospital policies and procedures, the participants will generally not have an extensive background of classroom and study experience. The approach to imparting information must alter to fit the needs of the students.

NURSE ATTENDANTS AND ORDERLIES

Role of the Nurse Attendant

Long before selecting content and deciding how to schedule it, examination of the roles and relationships of the health care team is necessary. Exactly what should nurse attendants be doing in your hospital? Has a job analysis ever been performed, or did the role gradually develop over the years with little or no guidance or direction? When an actual analysis of the nurse attendant job is done, the examiners are often shocked to discover that what is actually being done bears little resemblance to the formal job description. Sometimes the role varies from unit to unit, with one group of NAs performing basic nursing care and another group operating far outside legal boundaries, hanging bottles of intravenous fluid, performing sterile procedures, suctioning tracheotomy patients, and doing other tasks that should never have been delegated.

The nurses are at fault for allowing this to happen, particularly the managers. The tragedy is that although the nurse in charge is liable for any legal problems, so is the nurse attendant. Whoever performs a procedure is accountable for its effects, and this legal liability then proceeds up the chain of command under the legal doctrine of respondeat superior. How many NAs are working at inappropriate roles, unaware that they are open to lawsuits with potentially enormous settlements? If employees operate outside written policies, the hospital's legal representatives or the insurance company could win a judgment against those employees to recover some of the losses incurred in a lawsuit.

Protecting both patients and staff requires firm practice guidelines for all personnel—with follow-up by nursing administration to be sure the job descriptions are being followed. How does your hospital define the nurse attendant role? What tasks and procedures are appropriate for them to perform? How will you limit the role? Ideally, the role should be defined positively: a list of things that nurse attendants are able to do. Some policies may have to be stated in the negative—the "high-risk" procedures may require definite statements that nurse attendants may *not* . . . hang IVs, change sterile dressings, administer medications, perform sterile suctioning, etc.

Kramer and Schmalenberg have divided nursing care into two categories:

(1) inert tasks—those presenting a predictable amount of resistance that does not vary much over repeated performances;
(2) active tasks—those presenting an unpredictable and highly variable amount of resistance and which require decision making and judgment.[2]

Approaching task performance from this viewpoint, inert tasks would be appropriate for NAs to perform, while the highly variable active tasks require professional knowledge and judgment to assess and deal with the amount of resistance likely to occur. Kramer and Schmalenberg feel that often work is assigned on the basis of surface characteristics rather than the amount of variability and resistance; delegating active tasks to auxiliary workers results in a greater margin of error while assigning professional nurses to inert tasks can lead to inefficiency, lowered morale, and boredom.[3]

Task analysis can reveal what patient care tasks have little resistance (inert), such as bedmaking, and which are highly variable (active), such as patient teaching. One word of warning: some of these decisions may be quite controversial. Kramer and Schmalenberg feel that 90 percent of medication administration is inert, for example, while ambulating a postoperative patient for the first time is highly active.[4] Obviously, such division of tasks must be settled by consensus in a series of meetings—a major task for nursing administration, but perhaps one that is long overdue.

Some hospitals have added a category of "Senior Nurse Attendant" or some other title denoting a step up from basic NA performance. These long-term employees are often allowed expanded responsibilities as a method of motivation or reward for long service. The potential for allowing too much leeway in the role is enormous. The cheapest and easiest way to overcome this difficulty is not to create such a category in the first place. If the decision is made to have senior NAs, one way to develop the role is to assign these employees to work with a nurse in a "partner" relationship. Working side by side, the nurse and NA can provide excellent care by extending the nurse's range with an extra pair of hands and by demonstrating assessment and decision making for the NA.

Role of the Orderly

Male nurse attendants are often called orderlies. In some hospitals orderlies have the same responsibilities as any NA, but many institutions require orderlies to perform special tasks such as male catheterization. Such role variations require specialized training and clinical follow-up. Preparing a class on male catheterization, for instance, means presenting a review of pertinent anatomy and physiology, the theory of catheterizing patients, a demonstration of the procedure, and then allowing return demonstrations until the orderly displays consistently high performance.

Such a class then must be reinforced in the clinical area by supervised practice and follow-up, including periodic spot checks. Allowing a nonprofessional worker to perform such potentially dangerous procedures is risky, and the legal liability embraces orderly, instructor, team leader, nurse manager, and hospital. Are orderlies performing extremely active tasks based on a job description developed during a nursing shortage, or because it is expedient? Neither of those reasons is viable. In settings where no orderlies are available, female nurses catheterize male patients and no one thinks anything about it. The role of orderly needs careful scrutiny, with a decision based on patient needs.

Orienting Experienced Nurse Attendants and Orderlies

Assessment

Hospitals that hire only people with experience can present a shorter orientation program with the assumption that the new employees have a foundation of knowledge and experience to build on. This assumption may be faulty. Careful assessment of the orientee's background is vital. If pre-employment tests are used as a basis for hire, such tests must be validated by having a large sample of current NAs take them, performing an item analysis, and creating tests that a majority of the people working in the job category can pass. Then the tests must be given to all applicants, using the same standards for hire. Even with these safeguards, pre-employment tests can be challenged by disappointed applicants. It is safer to base hiring decisions on other factors and save the testing for orientation.

Assessment of knowledge and experience should be a mixture of written examinations and performance tests. Rather than relying on theory questions, base tests on practical, experiential matters. Give the new NAs patient situations and ask them how they would chart in those situations. Check knowledge of theory through questions such as those in Exhibit 12–1. While in-depth knowledge of physiology is not necessary to answer these, they do require the orientee to understand basic concepts of intake and output.

Selection of Content

Content selection must be based on job description and responsibilities of the NA in your institution. The results of individual assessment may influence your

---

Exhibit 12–1 NA Orientation Test

Intake and Output

What areas contribute to a patient's fluid intake?

____
____
____

What areas contribute to a patient's output? (What is measured?)

____
____
____
____

What might influence a patient's total fluid output?

____
____
____
____
____

Source: Education Department, Huntington Memorial Hospital, Pasadena, California. Reprinted with permission.

approach to the content, but the basic curriculum can be planned in advance by determining what information and practice is required to perform the role correctly.

Actual class content starts with program objectives. After determining the role and job responsibilities of the NA, ask what the orientees will be expected to do at the end of orientation. Based on these expectations, overall program objectives can be written to guide class selection (see Exhibit 12–2). When these objectives are reviewed on the first day of orientation, the orientees have a clear idea of what will be presented and what they are responsible for accomplishing within the set time frame.

Exhibit 12–2 NA Orientation Objectives

By the end of the two-week orientation, the new nurse attendant should be able to:

1. badge in and badge out correctly.
2. complete an exception report in an accurate manner.
3. provide care for a full assignment of patients, including A.M./P.M. care; bed baths, tub baths, or showers; safe ambulation; range-of-motion exercises; proper positioning; pre- and post-operative care; accurate vital signs; and accurate intake and output.
4. Correctly and completely document the following on the chart:
   a. At least one complete admission, including the Admission Sheet and the Admission note on the Nurses' Clinical Record.
   b. At least one discharge, including each of the five required pieces of information about the discharge.
   c. Nurses' notes for several complete shifts on a number of patients, with everything that was done for the patient written, as well as all observations about the patient.
   d. Any urine testing (C/A) on the Diabetic Record.
   e. All intake and output recorded on the bedside sheet and on the Intake/Output record.
   f. A.M./P.M. care, bath, and ambulation progress on the Graphic Sheet.
5. Care for at least one isolation patient, demonstrating double-bagging technique, correct handwashing and gowning, and complete documentation of patient care.
6. Transfer at least one patient from bed to chair and back again, demonstrating good body mechanics, safely supporting the patient, and correctly judging how much help is needed (if any).
7. Document food intake of all patients cared for, including percent taken and how tolerated, using correct charting procedure.
8. Keep team leader informed of patient progress throughout the day, with a complete report given at the end of the shift.
9. Empty all output containers after measuring at the end of the shift, and record on the Intake/Output Record.
10. Report any patient/family requests or complaints promptly to the proper person.

Source: Education Department, Huntington Memorial Hospital, Pasadena, California. Reprinted with permission.

The length of the program is determined by the individual institution and its needs, as well as by program objectives. Typically, an orientation program for experienced NAs is one to two weeks long. Exhibit 12–3 is a sample of such an orientation schedule. Besides showing the orientees what will be happening to them in the coming weeks, this serves as a communication tool between instructor and unit. The clinical days have a description of what the orientee should be doing—buddy system in the first week so that the new NA can "learn the ropes," then gradually increasing patient assignments until a full patient load is achieved. Theoretically, this would be accomplished by the end of the second week for experienced NAs, at which time they would go to permanent shift assignment and be considered full staff members. But in reality, not all orientees will follow this plan. The unit manager and clinical instructor may determine that a certain NA needs more supervised experience before completing orientation.

Methods of Classroom Presentation

Some NA orientees have little experience with classwork; indeed, some of their past school experiences may have been negative. If they are forced to sit in a classroom for eight hours listening to an instructor lecture, those negative experiences may rise up and block learning. This is not to say that lecture cannot be used. Richardson feels that lecture and role modeling are good ways to transmit desired attitudes to NAs, but demonstration/return demonstration/supervised practice are necessary when motor skills must be learned quickly.[5]

Obviously, a mixture of teaching techniques will be most effective with this group of learners, as with any group. For instance, discussion is a good strategy to begin with; discussing the role of the NA in the health care team involves learners immediately and enables the instructor to discover the experiences, knowledge, and values of the participants. Exhibit 12–4 outlines one way to lead from a general discussion of roles and responsibilities to a discussion of the specific duties of the NA.

One problem area in NA orientation concerns charting. Proper documentation of care requires the caregiver to write a description of patient appearance, concerns, and activities. If someone has difficulty with vocabulary, syntax, spelling—even poor handwriting—charting can be jeopardized. When working with NAs who have previous hospital experience, it is not unreasonable to assume that they already know the mechanics of charting. It is not unreasonable—but it may be unrealistic. Some institutions do not allow auxiliary workers to chart at all, requiring the nurses to complete all documentation. Not only does this increase the work of already overburdened nurses, the legality of charting something that one did not actually do or see done is extremely shaky. If challenged, the nurses could not truthfully state that the care they charted was done, only that they were told it was done (or worse, that they assumed it was done).

Exhibit 12–3 NA Orientation Schedule

Orientee: ______________________ Head Nurse: ______________________
Unit: ______________________ Orientation Instructor ______________________

Monday	Tuesday	Wednesday	Thursday	Friday
8:00–4:30 EDUC. DEPT. 8:00–2:30 New Employee Orient. 2:30–4:30 Unit (Observation)	8:00–4:30 EDUC. DEPT. Nursing Orientation Classes	7:00–3:30 UNIT Buddy System	8:00–4:30 EDUC. DEPT. 8:00–11:00 New Employee Orient. 11:00–11:45 Lunch 11:45–4:30 NA Orientation	7:00–3:30 UNIT Buddy System
8:00–4:30 EDUC. DEPT. Nursing Orientation Classes	7:00–3:30 UNIT Patient Care for 4 patients	7:00–3:30 UNIT Patient Care for 6 patients	7:00–3:30 UNIT Patient Care (Full patient assignment)	7:00–3:30 UNIT Patient Care (Full patient assignment) (GO TO UNIT SCHEDULE)

Source: Education Department, Huntington Memorial Hospital, Pasadena, California. Reprinted with permission.

Exhibit 12–4 Sample Outline from NA Orientation

I. Review objectives
II. The team and patient care
  A. How does a nursing team work?
  B. What experiences have you had working as a team member?
    1. What makes a good day?
    2. If problems arise, how can they be handled?
  C. What is the role of the head nurse?
III. Routine and responsibilities of the NA
  A. Review a typical day's schedule on the unit.
  B. Discuss the following:
    1. AM Care (What is it? When is it done?)
    2. Daily diet report, mealtimes, feeding patients (What is the NA responsible for?)
    3. What do you do at bathtime besides the bath?
      a. Linen change
      b. Range of motion exercises
      c. Observations (examples)
      d. Talking with the patient (Why is this important?)
      e. Position changes
      f. Cleaning room (straightening up, wiping off overbed table, etc. Can you think of an instance when you would want to be careful how you rearranged the room or table?).

Since forbidding NAs to chart is obviously not the answer, provide plenty of charting practice in class. Exhibit 12–5 shows an excerpt from an NA orientation class. One of the charting situations is described in Exhibit 12–6. All such patient situations should be written from the point of view of the nurse attendant, rather than the nurse-oriented viewpoints often found in textbooks. Write cases describing your setting and your patients, in order to make them meaningful and useful for the orientees.

Another area of weakness concerns accurate recording of intake and output. Although this problem is unfortunately not limited to auxiliary workers, they are often the caregivers most involved with this vitally important area. Discussions about accurate reports and the crucial information that intake and output records give physicians must always be included in orientation. Plenty of classroom practice helps develop the basic mathematical skills needed and provides opportunities to discuss the implications of the data recorded (see Exhibit 12–7).

Clinical Follow-up

Although some review of equipment and procedures is necessary in NA classes, the bulk of procedures review and practice for an experienced group of participants

Exhibit 12–5 Excerpt from NA Orientation Class

V. How do you communicate the information you collect?
   A. Team leader
      1. AM report
      2. Report at end of shift
      3. How can you keep the team leader informed between these two set times?
   B. Charting
      1. Why is documentation important?
      2. What should be written?
      3. Have you had any problems communicating the patients' needs and reactions?

VI. Charting Practice
   A. Nurses' Notes
      1. Give patient situations for practice.
      2. Chart instructor's version on board and have participants compare their versions with it.
      3. Discuss reasons for charting that way and other ways it could have been recorded.
      4. Give other situations that participants have had problems with in the past.
   B. Diabetic Record
      1. Practice charting urine testing results.
      2. Discuss problem of false positives.
      3. Stress importance of verbally reporting results as well as charting them.

Exhibit 12–6 Patient Situation from NA Charting Practice

Mr. J. is supposed to have X-rays tomorrow. You are supposed to give him three tap water enemas this evening. After dinner you go in to begin. He has only eaten a buttered roll and milk for supper. When you ask about that, he says, "I just don't feel very hungry tonight." You explain about the enemas, position him, and begin. After taking about 200 cc. of the enema, the patient begins to moan. You stop the flow and ask what's wrong. He says he's having some cramps, but to go ahead and "get this over with." You turn the flow back on very slowly, but after 50 cc. more have gone in he suddenly says, "I can't hold any more!" As you withdraw the tube, a lot of black, foul-smelling liquid stool spurts all over Mr. J. and the bed. While you help him wash and get him fresh linen he keeps crying to himself and saying, "I'm just like a little baby. I'm no good to anyone like this."

What would you report to the nurse? When?

Write down exactly how you would chart what happened.

Exhibit 12–7 Intake and Output Practice

Intake (10–6)		Output (10–6)	
1 glass H_2O	________	Foley DC at 11 P.M.	
1 glass cranberry juice	________	50 cc	
1 can soda pop	________	75 cc	
		50 cc	
Total	________	Total	________

Would you be concerned about the above intake and output? If so, why?

____

____

____

____

____

____

____

Source: Education Department, Huntington Memorial Hospital, Pasadena, California. Reprinted with permission.

will be done in the clinical area. This means that someone must work closely with each orientee to be sure procedures are performed correctly and unit policies and routines are followed. Usually this is handled by assigning a staff NA to each orientee as a buddy; these two work together for a few days before the orientee receives an individual patient assignment. If staff assigned to the buddy system are excellent performers with high morale and good attitudes, this approach should work well. If not, their influence on impressionable orientees can wreak incalculable damage.

Why not assign new attendants to work side by side with an RN or LPN? The professional nurse can validate orientee performance while providing an excellent role model. Taking this approach one more step, perhaps the outmoded team system could be replaced with a primary care approach that includes auxiliary workers. In settings where there simply are not enough nurses to properly implement true primary care, assigning a nurse attendant as partner (as described in the case of senior attendants in the section on roles) could provide better care, more job satisfaction, higher productivity, and promote a much closer team feeling than team nursing ever did.

Validation of performance should include not only observation of performance, but periodic paper and pencil tests as well. Exhibit 12–8 shows sample questions from such a test. Other questions might cover charting situations, cases calling for judgments on what should be reported, policy questions, etc.

Exhibit 12–8 Excerpt from NA Examination

Intake (6–2)		Output (6–2)	
1 pot coffee	________	Foley—650 cc	
1 glass H_2O	________		
½ glass juice	________		
⅓ glass H_2O	________		
¼ carton milk	________		
½ dish jello	________		
Total	________	Total	________

Intake (2–10)		Output (2–10)	
1 cup soup	________	Foley—100 cc	
1 cup tea	________		
½ cup custard	________		
⅔ glass juice	________		
1 cup tea	________		
Total	________	Total	________

What would you check before reporting these totals to the team leader?

____

____

____

____

____

____

Source: Education Department, Huntington Memorial Hospital, Pasadena, California. Reprinted with permission.

Orienting People With No Experience

The reasons for hiring inexperienced people (laypeople, in effect) as nurse attendants usually relate to that very inexperience. Some hospitals feel that such people will have no bad habits to unlearn and can be molded into the type of nurse attendants wanted by hospital managers. While this may hold true during the orientation period, the theory ignores the impact of the work environment when orientation is over. Peer pressure and modeling probably play a much more important part in the ultimate outcome than does initial training.

Rowland and Rowland state that "if unskilled workers are employed as nurse attendants who will be involved in direct patient services, they must be provided with on-the-job skill training. They must be taught the knowledge and skills required to perform their defined functions, with measures taken to safeguard the quality of nursing care."[6] What are these skills—and how can you build in the required safeguards?

Since the skills needed by nurse attendants in your institution have been identified by the job analysis previously discussed, the important decision that now must be made concerns the background knowledge required to function safely in the NA role. Should these learners receive information about basic anatomy and physiology? How much knowledge about the rationales for the different procedures should they have? Potentially, such a course could last for many weeks of eight-hour class days. A balance must be struck between what these participants need to know and the potential deluge of "nice to know" information.

The costs of these basic preparatory programs are persuading many hospitals to discontinue them. In some communities, vocational schools and community colleges offer sound basic NA preparatory programs, with the graduates hired by area hospitals. Other institutions hire only nursing students as attendants, thereby ensuring a solid foundation of theory. This strategy also serves as a recruitment tool.

Self-Study Programs

Several hospitals have tried self-study programs for nurse attendant orientation with some success. The approach described by Boyer is to hire only experienced NAs and base their orientation on:

1. An individual assessment determined through testing
2. Organizational needs
3. Validation of five commonly performed skills.[7]

Self-study packages are used to remedy only identified deficiencies, and nurse attendant orientation is usually accomplished in five days.[8]

A similar program is described by Kircher, in which self-study packages are assigned to orientees on the basis of written and performance testing results. The self-instructional packages cover tasks such as applying antiembolism stockings, with actual equipment and basic information packaged into each module. Learning is measured by written test, one in each package.[9] Some information, such as CPR, fire safety, and transfer techniques is presented by videotape. Task practice and written examinations measure the effectiveness of these classes.[10]

Validation of clinical performance is especially important with a self-study system. Prolonged work with a buddy may be required, or instructors, managers, and staff can use performance checklists to evaluate the orientees. In one hospital, head nurses were asked to assign a priority rating to the functions of NAs. The top five procedures were written as performance checklists, with critical elements of the task starred. Then any member of the nursing team familiar with the procedure could check off performance with a new employee. The performance of 24 of 28 attendants has been validated this way, with little or no additional cost and without disrupting unit work flow.[11]

Self-study programs can be used effectively but time and money must be spent planning, constructing, and implementing them. Careful assessment of each individual orientee is also essential if this process is to be successful. If people are hired who have difficulty with self-study, the program will discriminate against their chances for success. Will your NA candidates be familiar with the study skills and self-discipline required for such a program? A pilot program could provide the answer.

Special Preparation for Attendants and Orderlies

Some hospitals offer special programs to expand the role of nurse attendants and orderlies. With additional training, these workers become orthopedic technicians, for example, responsible for setting up traction apparatus. Others may work in labor and delivery, caring for instruments, sterilizing and stocking equipment and supplies. Exhibit 12–9 is a job description for such a technician.

Participants for such a program must be carefully selected. They have to be able to handle the advanced training and increased responsibilities of the role. Legal problems such as those mentioned in connection with the position of "senior nurse attendants" can occur with these special jobs. New job descriptions must be written to minimize liability, and the nurses must be willing to accept the increased responsibility they will have to supervise the attendants operating in an expanded role.

Considering the costs and risks of such programs, each hospital must decide if the benefits outweigh the potential risks. Perhaps the money might be better spent hiring more nurses. Make the decision based on patient needs rather than an automatic response to staff shortages or budget problems.

UNIT SECRETARY ORIENTATION

Unit secretaries perform invaluable services for the health care team. Since the role was developed, unit secretaries (or ward clerks, as they are often called) have taken on many of the clerical duties that prevented nurses from giving direct patient care. Unit secretaries now complete forms, answer phones, stock and order supplies, record vital signs on the chart, arrange admissions and discharges, and transcribe physicians' orders. These increased responsibilities benefit the direct care givers and thus the patients, but they also make the job of unit secretary one of the most difficult in the hospital.

Exhibit 12–9 Labor and Delivery Technician Job Description

Summary of Duties

Under the supervision of a registered nurse, the technician performs listed patient care tasks, cleans and restocks the delivery rooms, cleans, packs, and sterilizes instrument packs.

Job Responsibilities

1. When directed by the nurse in charge, administers perineal preps and tap water enemas to admitted patients who have been examined by a physician.
2. Takes oral temperatures, pulse rates, respirations, and blood pressures on patients in normal labor.
3. With the aid and instruction of a registered nurse, helps transfer patients from bed to stretcher and from stretcher to delivery table.
4. After the patient has been transferred to the recovery area, cleans the delivery room according to proper procedure, restocking all tables, drawers, and equipment areas.
5. Cleans instruments, forceps, baby packs, etc., arranges them in proper order according to the procedure book, and sterilizes each for the proper length of time.
6. Conducts the sterilizer test each morning, using test materials to ensure proper autoclave function and filing the record in the proper notebook.
7. Folds the clean linen delivered by the Laundry shortly after it comes up (depending on work load), following the procedure book instructions for proper methods of folding towels, drapes, leggings, sheets, etc.
8. Restocks supplies in utility room and autoclave room as needed. Reports stock and equipment to be ordered in a timely fashion.
9. Checks the contents of all emergency carts and all caesarean section carts daily for outdated supplies and packs. Resterilizes/restocks as necessary to keep all carts current.
10. Checks labor rooms after Housekeeping personnel have cleaned them, and restocks as necessary. Checks and restocks unused labor rooms at the beginning of each shift.
11. Assists registered nurses with patient care as directed, including assisting with emergency deliveries or CPR.

Preparation Required

One week of special classes after completing orientation for hospital nurse attendants. CPR training mandatory.

Orienting unit secretaries presents special problems, since the role covers so many different responsibilities. A person with experience in an ordinary secretarial position would find little of the background helpful. Most hospitals either hire experienced unit secretaries, train nurse attendants in the role, or take talented laypeople and train them from scratch. Whatever the approach, the orientees must learn what a unit secretary can and cannot do, as well as the awesome legal liability that accompanies the role.

Role of the Unit Secretary

Perhaps the most important aspect of the unit secretary's role is that of liaison for the nursing team. The secretaries serve as conduits of information to and from patients, visitors, physicians, members of other departments, and the nurses. For many people the first contact they have with the unit is the secretary. An attitude of concern is crucial. Can it be taught in orientation? Or must the personal qualities be discovered during hiring interviews? No simple answer exists, but the implications for the instructor are clear: orientation must teach not only skills but attitudes.

Other responsibilities of unit secretaries may include clerical ones such as filing, arranging charts in discharge order, and handling requisitions and other forms, and clinical ones such as taking wheelchair patients down for discharge or performing CPR in an emergency. All of this must be covered in orientation, depending on the job description in the particular institution. A unique responsibility is that of transcribing physicians' orders. This time-consuming task, handled by unit secretaries in most hospitals, is not only tedious but includes an enormous potential for serious errors. During orientation the new unit secretaries must learn not only how to accurately and completely transcribe orders but also the legal implications for them, the patients, nurses, and physicians.

Selection of Content

Program content is based on hospital philosophy and the unit secretary job description, but this is one program where the content will vary little for the experienced versus the inexperienced participant. Although prior experience in the role is helpful, policies and procedures differ so greatly from hospital to hospital that even the experienced person must learn the job from the ground up. If assessment testing is used after hire, it may indicate areas that need extra emphasis, such as telephone or filing skills, but the basic content should be covered for all participants.

Exhibit 12–10 is an example of overall program objectives for a unit secretary orientation. The length of this particular program is three weeks, with job candidates screened carefully for ability, stable prior employment, and maturity. No one is hired directly from school; while unit secretary experience is not required, some job must have been held before.

Classwork and clinical experience should be mixed together for unit secretary orientation. With job duties so eclectic and complex, a unit secretary must have frequent practice and reinforcement in the clinical area, or information covered in class will be lost. Exhibit 12–11 shows a typical orientation day demonstrating this mix, unit experience alternating with classroom work.

Exhibit 12–10 Program Objectives for US Orientation

Unit Secretary Orientation

Purpose: This program is designed to introduce the new Unit Secretary to his/her job functions, provide an understanding of the Unit work flow, and the physical layout of Huntington Memorial Hospital.

Objectives: Upon completion of the orientation program, the Unit Secretary will be able to perform the following:

- all applicable CRT functions
- transcription and initiation of physician orders
- patient admit, transfer, and discharge process
- utilization of patient chart and forms
- independent and confidential functioning with procedures relating to the Unit, patient, and public

Source: Systems Planning and Development Department, Huntington Memorial Hospital, Pasadena, California. Reprinted with permission.

Clinical Follow-Up

The only person who can teach a unit secretary exactly what to do and how to do it is another unit secretary. Although classroom theory is important and necessary, the orientee really learns how to put the information together and use it while working with an experienced unit secretary in the clinical area. Preceptors should be chosen not merely for their expertise but also for a willingness and ability to share that expertise. A staff member who doesn't like to work with new people can crush an orientee's morale and motivation faster than any class or pep talk can bolster them.

Evaluation of new unit secretaries should be carefully planned from the beginning of the program. Involve all key personnel, particularly the preceptor and head nurse. Methods of evaluation will be covered in detail in Chapter 13, but unit secretary assessment must cover more than the activities and behaviors of the orientee. That intangible called "attitude" figures prominently in the unit secretary role and must be appraised also. The manager sets standards for answering the phone, for example: "The unit secretary must respond with:

1. Unit name
2. Unit secretary's name
3. The phrase, 'May I help you?'"

Exhibit 12–11 US Orientation Schedule

Date/Time	*Content*	*Responsibility*	*Shifts*
Tuesday-Week I	(Check In/Out on Unit CRT)		
0700–0845	Unit Observation and Assistance Continuation of prior Monday	New Employee with Unit Assistance	Days and P.M.S
0845–0900	Break		
0900–1100	I. Utilization of computer generated reports A. Rental Sheet B. Diet Report C. Med Records D. Daily Patient Information Sheet E. Day/Night Sheet F. TPR II. Patient admitting procedures III. Transcribing doctors' orders IV. Cardex utilization	Systems Planning and Development	Days and P.M.S
1100–1230	Tour of: A. Clinical Lab B. Cashier/Front Desk C. Dismissal Area D. CSS E. Dispensary F. Stat Lab G. Outpatient Pharmacy H. Nursing Administration I. Medical Records	Systems Planning and Development	Days and P.M.S
1230–1300	Lunch		
1300–1500	CRT Class I Instruction of CRT functions	Systems Planning and Development	Days and P.M.S
1500–1530	Unit Observation and Assistance Continuation of prior Monday	New Employee with Unit Assistance	Days and P.M.S

Source: Systems Planning and Development Department, Huntington Memorial Hospital, Pasadena, California. Reprinted with permission.

But what about the tone of voice in which the correct statements are made? Documentation of a bored or surly response rather than politeness or enthusiasm can be followed by counseling and, hopefully, improvement.

Self-Study Programs

Boyer describes a self-study program for unit secretaries where orientees complete self-learning packages and then practice the skills on the unit with a preceptor. The training takes four weeks, with minimal instructor time, as opposed to the previous six-week course that had been used, which required many hours of classwork. Advantages include the ability to hire and orient a unit secretary at any time, immediate application of learning, and increased cost effectiveness.[12]

Unit secretaries are ideal participants for self-study programs, since an effective unit secretary must be able to quickly assimilate the written word. And they seem to be more internally motivated than some other categories of workers. Exhibit 12–12 shows a sample page from a self-study workbook for unit secretaries. The procedures for each area impacting on the unit secretary can be included in such a self-study tool. The workbook is always available for reinforcement, and performance can be practiced and validated with the clinical preceptor.

Games and puzzles can be used to present information in an entertaining way. Exhibit 12–13 is an example of crossword puzzle format used to review information covered in the self-study section on health care law. Including the answers at the back of the workbook enables orientees to validate their responses themselves (see Exhibit 12–14), or answers could be provided by the preceptor or instructor.

With a self-study program, evaluation becomes doubly important. The instructor loses the chance to observe orientees in class and so must rely wholly on observations and performance appraisals from the clinical area. Besides the action analyses done by instructors and unit personnel, periodic written examinations help keep orientees and staff aware of progress and final accomplishments. Short check point quizzes can be included at the end of each section of the self-study workbook, with a final examination upon completion. Exhibit 12–15 is an excerpt from such a test. Note that it can be removed from the notebook and turned in for grading.

If an evaluation is included at the back of the self-study workbook (see Exhibit 12–16), orientees can give feedback on the format and information so that changes can be incorporated in response to learner reactions. Question number 9 is especially pertinent, since it gears feedback to actual on-the-job performance.

Exhibit 12–12 Page from Self-Study Workbook for US

SECURITY

LOST AND FOUND

Take valuables (money, jewelry, glasses, dentures) to the Nursing Service Administration Office. Take clothing and personal belongings to the Housekeeping Department.

LOSS OR DAMAGE TO PERSONAL PROPERTY

The procedure for reporting loss of property belonging to a patient, visitor or employee is as follows:

A. Telephone Administration Department. If closed call the Nursing Service Administration Office (Nursing Office).

B. Telephone Safety and Security Department.

C. Complete a "Report of Loss, Damage to Personal Property" (Form #RN 7660). If the loss of property belongs to a patient, the form should be completed by the person to whom it was reported by the Nurse-in-Charge. Send any report involving loss to a patient directly to the Nursing Administration Office.

KEYS

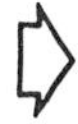

Only authorized personnel (approved in writing by the Department Head) may receive keys. To order keys complete a "Work Order Request" (form 62620); obtain signature of Department Head; and send form to Maintenance Department. When a new key is received, the Department Head or authorized employee signs the "Work Accepted By" section of the form.

Source: Education Department, Hospital of the Good Samaritan, Los Angeles, California. Reprinted with permission.

Exhibit 12–13 Crossword Puzzle Format Used in Workbook

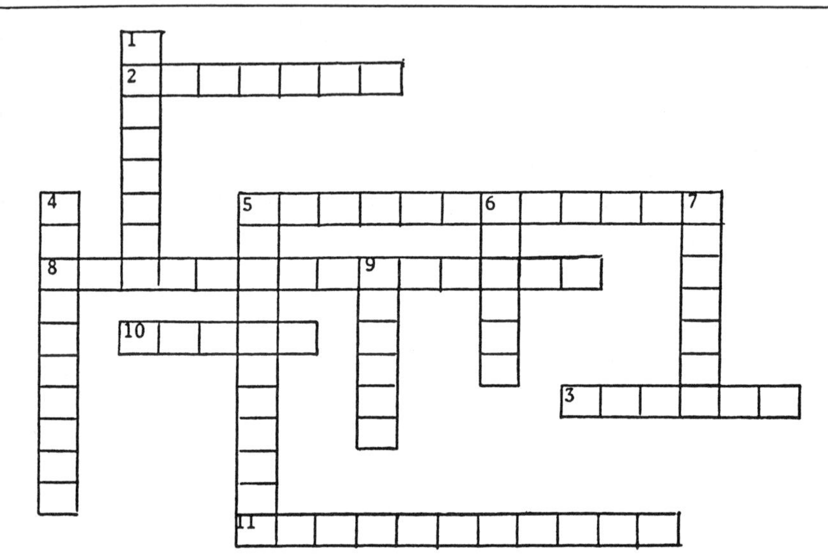

ACROSS

2 = Is what you can give a patient to eat or drink
3 = The only person allowed to answer questions a patient has about illness or treatment
5 = Describes how you treat all information about patients
8 = Ethical laws explaining what hospitals can and cannot do to patients (2 words)
10 = Is how often you help move or lift a patient
11 = Negligence of <u>any</u> hospital employee which may cause injury to a patient

DOWN

1 = What happens to other people when you don't observe safety practices
4 = Who you ask when you don't know how to handle a patient
5 = A form which a patient signs to give a hospital the right to treat him/her (2 words)
6 = Moral principles guiding individual actions
7 = What a patient may do when s/he's not happy with our service
9 = What is done in writing for any and all incidents

Source: Education Department, Hospital of the Good Samaritan, Los Angeles, California. Reprinted with permission.

Exhibit 12–14 Answer Sheet to Crossword Puzzle (Exhibit 12–13)

ACROSS

2 = Nothing

3 = Doctor

5 = Confidential

8 = Patients Rights

10 = Never

11 = Malpractice

DOWN

1 = Incident

4 = Supervisor

5 = Consent Form

6 = Ethics

7 = Lawsuit

9 = Report

Source: Education Department, Hospital of the Good Samaritan, Los Angeles, California. Reprinted with permission.

Exhibit 12–15 Excerpt from US Examination

8. If you want more than 50 copies of an original, it is cheaper to use:
   a. The copy machine in your department.
   b. Copying service in Forms Management.
9. A repair request for changing a light bulb should be sent to:
   a. Biomedical Engineering
   b. Plant Operations/Maintenance
   c. Housekeeping
10. A request for repairing a beeper should be sent to:
   a. Biomedical Engineering
   b. Plant Operations/Maintenance
   c. Housekeeping
11. Which of the following publications contains changes in hospital policy?
   a. Informal Bulletin
   b. Direct Line
   c. Weekly Bulletin
12. Outside calls are transferred to another department by:
   a. You
   b. The hospital operator
   c. The telephone company
13. After filling out a "Repair/Work Order Request," you keep the:
   a. White copy
   b. Pink copy
   c. Yellow copy
14. Lost items of value (jewelry, money) should be taken to the:
   a. Nursing Administration Office
   b. Accounting Department
   c. Housekeeping Department
15. A short letter (100 words or less) should be:
   a. single-spaced between sentences
   b. double-spaced between sentences
   c. triple-spaced between sentences
16. The emergency number for reporting a Code Red, Code Blue or Triage is:
   a. #6
   b. #0
   c. #411

Source: Education Department, Hospital of the Good Samaritan, Los Angeles, California. Reprinted with permission.

Exhibit 12–16 US Self-Study Workbook Evaluation

Please help improve future editions of this manual by completing this questionnaire. Return to Education Department (Allied).

A. CONTENT (Circle one number on the continuum below.)

	OK				NOT OK	
1. Related to Job	5	4	3	2	1	Not Related
2. New Information	5	4	3	2	1	Old hat
3. Easy to Understand	5	4	3	2	1	Ambiguous
4. Helpful to Me	5	4	3	2	1	Not Helpful
5. Interesting	5	4	3	2	1	Boring
6. Organized	5	4	3	2	1	Disorganized

7. I would like to see the following information included in a future edition of this manual: ______________________________

____

____

8. I recommend the following changes to improve the manual:

____

____

____

9. Reading this manual has helped me to do a better job in the following areas:

__________ ______________________________

__________ ______________________________

____

Source: Education Department, Hospital of the Good Samaritan, Los Angeles, California. Reprinted with permission.

CONCLUSION

Auxiliary personnel support professional staff in care delivery, extending the nurses' ability to assess and administer patient care. Orientation programs for these workers offer background theory and task preparation, but only after a thorough examination of the roles and responsibilities. Through classwork, self-study, and closely supervised clinical experience, nonprofessional employees can learn to deliver safe, effective care, freeing the professionals to meet more complex patient needs.

NOTES

1. *Webster's Third New International Dictionary of the English Language, Unabridged, 17th Edition* (Chicago: Encyclopedia Britannica, 1976), 149.

2. Marlene Kramer and Claudia Schmalenberg, *Path to Biculturalism* (Wakefield, Mass.: Contemporary Publishing, 1977), 199.

3. Ibid., 200.

4. Ibid., 198–199.

5. Elizabeth Richardson, "Teaching Nursing Assistants," *Nursing Management* 13, no. 7 (July 1982): 36.

6. Howard S. Rowland and Beatrice L. Rowland, *Nursing Administration Handbook* (Rockville, Md.: Aspen Systems Corp., 1980), 229–230.

7. Catherine Boyer, "Performance-Based Staff Development: The Cost-Effective Alternative," *Nurse Educator* 6, no. 5 (September/October 1981): 13.

8. Ibid., 13.

9. Sue Kircher, "Aide Orientation," *Supervisor Nurse* 8, no. 10 (October 1977): 32.

10. Ibid., 32.

11. Ibid., 32–33.

12. Boyer, "Performance-Based Staff Development," 13.

Part IV

Evaluation

Chapter 13

Evaluation of Orientees

The dictionary defines *evaluate* as "to examine and judge concerning the worth, quality, significance, amount, degree, or condition of something."[1] When education is being evaluated, we generally think in terms of judging the effectiveness of the teaching and measuring what learning has occurred. But hospital education involves larger goals than merely learning for learning's sake. Tobin, Yoder-Wise, and Hull state that "the ultimate goal of the staff development process is performance directed toward maintenance of or improvement in the quality of patient care."[2] In planning and implementing evaluation of orientees and of the orientation program as a whole, hospital educators must focus on the quality of patient care as well as the short-term goals of learning and retention.

INSTRUCTOR RESPONSIBILITIES

Although performance appraisals are a management responsibility, instructors must evaluate student performance for the following reasons:

1. To determine if participants are assimilating information as it is being taught.
2. To determine if participants remember information after it has been taught.
3. To determine if participants can use the information in their day-to-day job performance.

There are two basic approaches to student evaluation: (1) *norm* performance tests, which compare each student with an established norm group, enabling the instructor to rank each learner in relation to other learners (for example, the National League of Nursing examinations for nursing students); and (2) *criteria* performance methods, which enable the student's behaviors to be compared with the behavioral objectives describing desired target behaviors.[3] For the purposes of orientation, criteria performance methods are best, since participants should be evaluated on their ability to perform in the desired manner—comparisons with each other or some other group would be unnecessary.

The basis for evaluation must be the program objectives. They serve as the standards or criteria against which learning and performance can be measured. Since objectives are shared with orientees at the very beginning of the program, each student understands and accepts these standards before beginning classes and clinical experience. The importance of writing specific, clearly stated objectives becomes apparent during evaluation. When objectives are expressed as demonstrable behaviors, both instructor and orientee know exactly what outcomes are expected and how they will be measured.

Douglass and Bevis feel that evaluation can be successful only if both instructor and learner have the data necessary to assess the present situation and to structure additional experiences for achievement of the desired behavioral changes. They stress that the ultimate purpose of individual evaluation is to provide the learner with a guide for accomplishing a stated goal.[4] The essence of the evaluation process, then, is feedback, which motivates learning by validating that learners are on the right track or by identifying additional needed knowledge or skills.[5]

Evaluation should be viewed as a process intended to point out what is good as well as what needs to be corrected. Pohl stresses that educators should constantly remind themselves to appraise the *activity*, not the person.[6] This can be especially hard if the orientee's personality clashes with yours, but bringing personal characteristics into the evaluation process leads to hard feelings, low motivation, and lessened chances for improvement. The best way to ensure objectivity is to plan evaluation methods that are used for all orientees from the beginning of orientation to the end. A standard evaluation method encourages objective appraisal and progress reports on all orientees, not just ones perceived as "problem" employees.

METHODS OF ORIENTEE EVALUATION

The orientation instructor can discover valuable information about new employees through evaluation carried out while they are being oriented. Table 13–1 lists several methods that may prove useful. Note that all of these are designed for use by instructors. They do not take the place of the formal performance appraisal completed by each orientee's manager. While important data learned through these methods should be communicated to the unit manager and may be used in performance appraisals, the real purpose of this type of evaluation is to validate learning.

Table 13–1 Methods of Orientee Evaluation

Testing	*Classroom and Clinical Observation*	*Self-Evaluation*
Written examinations	Checklists	Open-ended form
Simulation tests	Rating scales	Discussion
Laboratory tests	Anecdotal notes	

Testing

A test may be defined as any systematic procedure that provides descriptive data on one or more people.[7] Tests must be designed to assess achievement of the desired behaviors described by the objectives, and test giving should be standardized enough to be used with different people and different groups. Well-constructed tests help instructors to:

1. Assess participant progress
2. Diagnose difficulties
3. Measure the effect of the chosen content
4. Determine the effectiveness of the methods and materials used in teaching.[8]

Testing in a work situation can cause problems, since the process poses a threat to workers' self-esteem. If test results are used as a diagnostic tool to help employees, and as a method of review and learning, much of the threat is defused. However, if the results are to be used for evaluation, reward, or punishment, this should be made clear from the beginning. With careful planning, orientees can be so well prepared for the testing situation through review, discussion, and self-study that tests actually increase confidence and motivation by promoting successful experiences.

Written Examinations

In traditional education programs, written examinations are used to measure learning and retention of information. Pretests attempt to discover what knowledge of the subject students bring with them into the program. The use of pretests was discussed in Chapter 2 as part of the needs assessment process. In some hospitals pretests are used in the hiring decision. In order to be employed, applicants must pass a test of job knowledge, such as medical terminology for unit secretaries or medical transcribers. Using tests for hiring can cause legal problems unless they are very carefully validated, since disappointed applicants can claim that the examination was biased or deliberately used to discriminate against them. Although the method for validating such a test was described in Chapter 2, it is safer to save tests until after hire.

Once an employee is on staff, tests can be used as a requirement for practice. In some hospitals, nurses must pass a pharmacology test before being allowed to pass medications. If they are unable to achieve a passing score they may be required to repeat the test, complete a self-study program, register for a pharmacology course, or work as a nurse attendant until the test is passed. After a certain number of attempts, a nurse who still cannot pass the examination may be terminated. If such a policy is chosen it should be stated to applicants before hire and no exceptions can be made. If the policy is circumvented for some promising orientee who has trouble taking tests, the entire process has been compromised and should not be used.

Classroom testing yields valuable information on how well orientees are keeping up with the onslaught of medical and other relevant information. Pretests can be used not only to assess prior knowledge but also to pique interest in content. If pretests are collected and retained by the instructor, the scores can be compared to post-test results to demonstrate that knowledge has been gained.

Segall et al. offer a system for analyzing pre- and post-test data using the same instrument:

> High errors on pretest; low on post test = probably a good question, shows change after instruction.
> Low errors on pretest; high on post test = either the item is ambiguous or else instruction was misleading.
> High errors on pretest; high on post test = poor item or unsuccessful teaching.
> Low errors on pretest; low on post test = probably too easy, should not have been in the course.[9]

There are several formats for written tests: multiple choice, completion, true-false, etc. Many references are available on constructing objective test questions; instructors unused to writing examinations should study the ins and outs of testing, and practice composing test items. The most important thing to remember about written test items is that they must assess achievement of stated objectives. Every objective must be tested in some way to validate accomplishment. Exhibit 13–1 shows some individual class objectives for a session on the organization of the nursing department. How could orientees be tested on this content? Because the objectives are so specific, they can be taken almost as stated and made into an examination. The only objective that needs restatement as a test item is number 3, which could be worded: "(a) List three nursing committees; (b) If you had

Exhibit 13–1 Orientation Objectives Suitable for Testing

Organization of the Nursing Department

After participating in the session on Nursing Department organization, the orientee will be able to:

1. sketch the organization of the Nursing Department in outline form, listing the chain of command.
2. name her/his head nurse, clinician, clinical specialist, supervisor, and director of nursing.
3. explain the committee structure of the Nursing Department and how changes are instituted.
4. describe the procedure to be followed when calling in sick.

composed a new nursing care plan or wanted to suggest a procedure change, what steps would you take to implement your idea?''

When planning orientation, decide how testing will be conducted. Will tests be given after each class? Will a single examination be given at the end of the program covering all content? Generally, a series of smaller tests will prove more effective and less stressful than one comprehensive examination. Most students will try harder to learn the content when they know a test is coming, so be sure to inform the participants that they will be tested.

One way to use tests for instruction is to include ''minitests'' within classes. After a segment of information has been presented, ask a few questions about the content, using overhead transparencies so that the answers can remain covered and then be disclosed after the group has had a chance to respond. Such testing can be used to reemphasize the key points of instruction. Participant responses also highlight instructional weaknesses or illogical organization of content. This approach is especially helpful when a large amount of information must be covered. Exhibit 13–2 shows a number of important objectives on intravenous therapy. Periodic questions would help break down the content into manageable segments and provide frequent review, as well as testing mastery of past information before moving on to new material.

Simulation Testing

Written tests are limited in their ability to assess judgment as well as priority setting and data gathering skills. Most clinical situations are too complex to fit neatly into a multiple choice. Simulation tests resemble reality in that actual situations can be written or acted out. Participants must choose an action to take in response to the simulated occurrence. Such tests can be as simple as the excerpts in Exhibit 13–3, requiring a factual response, or extremely long clinical problems

Exhibit 13–2 Intravenous Therapy Objectives

After participating in the session on IV Therapy, the orientee will be able to:

1. discuss the duties of the IV Team.
2. correctly complete the IV order sheet for the unit.
3. assemble equipment for an IV before calling the team.
4. list the responsibilities of the unit nurse in intravenous therapy.
5. identify an infiltration and state the steps to follow.
6. list five actions you might take if you discovered that an IV was not dripping.
7. state the first step to take for a leaking IV.
8. explain the method of maintaining a heparin lock.
9. demonstrate the setup for an IV piggyback with a:
   a. partial fill
   b. volutrol
10. list the type and frequency of observations needed during blood administration.
11. list the symptoms of a transfusion reaction and explain the steps to follow if one occurs.
12. demonstrate the use of the IV pumps.
13. state the standing orders to follow when a patient is receiving hyperalimentation.
14. chart the following:
    a. A new IV bottle added to the present line.
    b. 300cc left to be absorbed in the bottle at the end of your shift.
    c. Garamycin 80mg. in 100cc D5W IVPB.
    d. The IV has infiltrated—site in R forearm swollen and cold to touch.
    e. A patient receiving blood complains of chills and flank pain. (Chart your actions.)

Source: Education Department, Huntington Memorial Hospital, Pasadena, California. Reprinted with permission.

describing physical, emotional, and sociological data and requiring orientees to assess patient problems and select appropriate interventions.

Zufall found that since simulation tests are purposely designed to represent reality, students find them more relevant than conventional tests and tend to become more involved.[10] Simulations also provide an excellent review of material (as in Exhibit 13–3), thus reinforcing learning while testing it. To write a simulation, choose a real situation that requires critical thinking and demonstrates behaviors based on objectives. Assessment will be easier if the range of responses is limited, so try to keep the questions short.

Simulations can be presented as role plays, live or on videotape, requiring participants to critique the performers' responses to a situation or to propose what actions should be taken next. Videotaping students as they work through role play is another method of testing. After completing the simulation the orientees evaluate their performance in the situation, either alone, with an instructor, or with the entire group. A word of warning: some people find this kind of test extremely threatening and may either refuse to appear before the camera or become so paralyzed with anxiety that the test is invalidated.

Exhibit 13–3 Excerpt from Simple Simulation Test

Mr. J., a 68-year-old patient who was admitted to one of the regular units for treatment of abdominal discomfort, has been having assorted lab tests and x-rays during his stay. This morning you were getting ready to pass medications when you heard them call a Code Blue—on Mr. J.! Rolling the Stat Cart down to the room, you find several people already giving CPR and turning the bed around. Helping them put the board under the patient, you put down the esophageal airway. A respiratory therapist rushes in and begins ventilating the patient, and out of the corner of your eye you notice the IV nurse has started an IV with 500 cc. 5% D/W. As you apply the B/P cuff and pick up the record sheet, Dr. Wishner orders the first drug, which is . . . .

(PLEASE TURN THE PAGE)

SODIUM BICARBONATE

The doctor knows that the patient is now acidotic, and wants to give the $NaHCO_3$ to neutralize the acidosis and bring the blood back to its proper pH(7.35-7.45). A variation of only 0.4 of a pH unit in either direction can be fatal. Sodium bicarbonate also helps correct hyperkalemia, which a change in pH can aggravate.

The pharmacist has automatically prepared 5 prefilled syringes. Now he gives a 50mEq bolus (1 amp.) as ordered. This may be followed by another dose every 5-10 minutes, but it is wisest to plan the dosage according to blood pH readings, as it is easy to overcarbonate the patient. Of course, you're watching the one administering the drug to be sure they flush the IV line with saline between doses, as $NaHCO_3$ is incompatible with many drugs. If you knew that Mr. J. had COPD, be sure to tell the doctor, because this drug is dangerous for those patients.

The scope shows V-fib. As you're charging the defibrillator, the doctor orders a drug to enhance defibrillation . . . .

(PLEASE TURN THE PAGE)

Laboratory Testing

Laboratories have long been used to teach procedures to nursing students and hospital employees. Recently the concept of testing in a laboratory setting has been introduced. The same advantages of simulation testing accompany a laboratory setting: verisimilitude and built-in validity, since the test so closely resembles reality.

A typical laboratory test includes stations that each student rotates through. For instance, in a test of the ability to perform intravenous procedures, participants might find a setup for a piggyback that they would have to assemble; a manikin with an intravenous line that has infiltrated, with instructions to chart their findings and take the appropriate action; a dressing that needs changing; and an intravenous arm with equipment for inserting an intracath. Schneider recommends a checklist of some kind by which the evaluator can systematically check off each of the steps or elements comprising the procedure.[11]

Test Relevance

Zufall suggests increasing test relevance by asking the following questions:

1. Did the test represent a problem that the learner may encounter and did the material presented in the course help the learner to deal with it?
2. Were the questions in proportion to the importance of behavior that the course attempted to develop?[12]

Instructors tend to rely heavily on test results to justify orientation content and structure: "Look, the orientees were able to score such-and-such, which proves they are learning the material." Before claiming too much, remember that written tests in particular are easy for experienced test takers to "beat" by guessing the right answers. Also, the tests may measure memory rather than the ability to perform. Simulation and laboratory testing demonstrate more relevance using Zufall's questions, but the results are more negative than positive. As Tobin, Yoder-Wise, and Hull accurately point out, if individuals cannot perform in a simulated situation, they are not likely to be able to perform in the real situation—but acceptable performance in a simulated situation does not necessarily indicate an ability to perform well in the real situation.[13]

Observation of Orientee Behavior

Learning takes time to be assimilated, another drawback to immediate factual testing. Instructors also use observation as a way of assessing how well students grasp the information presented. Such observations can take place in the classroom or in the clinical area.

Classroom Observation

Assessing student participation and reaction during class is not only a time-honored tactic, it goes on continuously, whether purposefully or accidentally. Who asks questions in class, and do the questions indicate in-depth investigation of the content that has been presented or merely inattention? Which participants can rephrase concepts in their own words and apply them to stated problems? What body language is evident in the group? After 30 minutes with a group of orientees, most instructors have formed opinions about the personalities, abilities, and potential of every person in the room.

Unfortunately, not all such opinions are valid. If an orientee normally works nights and had to report to class at seven or eight in the morning, response to the content is likely to be sluggish at best. Yet at night this same person may be a dynamo of good judgment and productivity. If a particular participant's communication style clashes with that of the instructor, a label of "uncooperative" or "inattentive" may follow that participant far beyond the classroom. Yet another instructor might find the same person "refreshingly candid" or "quiet and thoughtful."

Since observation *will* take place in the classroom, how can an instructor minimize bias and personal opinion? While subjectivity cannot be completely avoided, systematic observations promote objective assessment. What behavior do you want students to exhibit? Why? What behaviors demonstrate that learning is taking place? Do participants realize this? If you expect orientees to take notes or to ask (or answer) questions, *tell them*. Sharing your expectations enables participants to understand the standards being used to judge their behavior. Most important, remember that you are judging the activity, not the person.[14]

If behavior exhibited in class seems significant and likely to impact on clinical performance, how can your observations be communicated to unit personnel? Conveying information likely to affect an employee's career over the telephone or over a cup of coffee in the cafeteria is neither professional nor effective, and is open to misinterpretation. A better way is through an orientation communication form such as is shown in Exhibit 13–4, similar to the one discussed in Chapter 8. When information is presented, the classroom instructor initials the appropriate area. Observations about each orientee are recorded in the progress notes. When employees reach the unit, the pertinent data is there on the sheet. Validation of performance is initialed by both the clinician and the orientee, enabling the form to serve as a record of orientation when placed in the employee's personnel file.

Clinical Observation

When observing clinical performance, uniform observation is even harder to achieve than in the classroom because of the number of evaluators and frequent ambiguity of standards. In one study, two supervisors simultaneously and separately observed nurses carrying out procedures four times. High interrater reliability was obtained only when the observations were simultaneous.[15]

Observation Guidelines

One way to promote effective evaluation is to use guidelines such as checklists and rating scales to direct observation of performance. Expected behaviors are listed by category on most checklists, as with the skills inventory. Unlike the skills inventory, however, evaluatory checklists are completed by independent observers rather than the orientee. The observers may be instructors, managers, precep-

Exhibit 13–4 One Method of Communicating Observations

R.N./L.V.N. ORIENTATION CHECKLIST

EMPLOYEE ______________________ ORIENTATION START DATE __________

TOPICS	INSTRUCTOR DATE/INITIALS	CLINICIAN DATE/INITIALS	EMPLOYEE DATE/INITIALS
I. GENERAL INFORMATION			
Hospital Philosophy			
Organization Structure			
Benefits			
Job Description			
Badge In/Badge Out			
Exception Reports			
Sick Calls			
Employee Policies			
Professional Liability			
II. NURSING UNIT			
Physical Layout			
Location of equipment/supplies			
Methods of assignment			
Time schedules			
Special requests			
Shift change reporting system			
Charting guidelines			
Kardex			
Discharge planning			
Pneumatic tube system			
Evaluations			
III. PATIENT CARE REPORTS			
Patient Charts			
Notification forms			
Medication Error Reports			
Responsibility releases			

Patient census/condition reports			
Discharge sheet			
Decubitus care form			
Code Blue report forms			
Surgery consent forms			
Pre-operative checklists			
IV. POLICIES/PROCEDURES			
Admissions			
Transfers			
Discharges			
Surgery (pre & post-operative care)			
Death			
Intake/Output			
Isolation/Infection Control			
Transcribing Physician Orders			
Blood Transfusions			
IV Therapy			
Medication Administration			
Narcotic Control			
Fire Procedure			
Evacuation/Disasters			
Code Blue Procedures			
Nursing Care Plans			
Suctioning			
Oxygen Administration			
Op-site/stomadhesive			
Feeding tubes			
Electrical Safety			

PROGRESS NOTES: ____________________

INSTRUCTOR: __________ CLINICIAN: __________ EMPLOYEE: __________

tors, or even other employees. Exhibit 13–5 shows an excerpt from such a checklist used in the clinical laboratory. Note that the wording is as specific as possible so that the only judgment the observer need make is whether the behaviors were or were not performed. Since this reports on the orientee's behavior only on one occasion, observations should be repeated more than once and patterns noted.

Rating scales are descriptions of varying degrees of achievement.[16] They generally contain such terms as "above average," "average," "below average" or "superior," "good," "acceptable," "unacceptable." Exhibit 13–6 shows a rating scale used to evaluate orientees in the clinical area. In this instrument numbers are used to represent different ratings. The definitions of the standards are described in detail at the end of the form.

The drawback with rating scales is the degree of subjectivity involved. What makes one person "average" and another "above average"? Detailed descriptions of the behaviors expected may minimize observer bias, but many people like to expand their judgments with further notes.

Some prefer describing the clinical situation and the orientee's behavior in narrative, anecdotal form. Subjective interpretation can be minimized by describing the exact behaviors observed, even directly quoting statements made by the orientee, patient, or other participants in the situation.

Anecdotal notes take time to record, especially if they must be made after the fact—a situation that can lead to memory problems and errors. In fact, Bailey and Claus describe the three major limitations of observation as (1) subjectivity, (2) the presence of an observer (a variable that may alter the situation), and (3) fragmentary reporting resulting from the problem of observing and recording information at the same time.[17]

Self-Evaluation

When a clear description of expected outcomes is presented to orientees, Tobin, Yoder-Wise, and Hull feel they can evaluate their own situation or behavior and then relate it to those expected outcomes.[18] At the end of the probation period, which in most hospitals is three months, the unit manager meets with the employee to give feedback on performance. The orientee should share in the discussion and try to make specific suggestions for improvement.

McKeachie states that feedback results in improvement only when at least three conditions are present:

1. You learn if you get *new* information from the feedback.
2. You must be *motivated* to change.
3. You must be given *alternatives*—different ways of behaving.[19]

Exhibit 13–5 Excerpt from Laboratory Checklist

AUTOBAC (continued)	ACCEPTABLE	DATE	INITIAL
4. Record daily QC organisms and wedge readings			
5. Standardize saline suspension and perform AB test			
6. Proper sequence of antimicrobial discs in the cuvette			
7. Replace/replenish discs properly			
8. Let discs warm up at RT for at least one hour before use.			
BACTEC BLOOD CULTURE:			
1. Perform visual screening of vials for +			
2. Screen blood culture vials daily using Bactec blood culture equipment			
3. Prepare stains for positive vials			
4. Prepare necessary paperwork and other steps for positive blood cultures			
5. Subculture DAY 1 and DAY 5 vials onto chocolate plates			
6. Prepare preliminary and final reports			
7. Prepare necessary steps for direct suscept.			
8. Perform and record daily performance test			
9. Record gas pressure and display light daily			
10. Change needles, clean, and send to CSS			
ANAEROBIC CHAMBER:			
1. Utilize anaerobic chamber -- glove ports and transfer module			
2. Process anaerobic specimen in chamber			
3. Disinfect and restock anaerobic chamber			
4. Reactivate catalysts			
5. Utilize gas pak jars			
6. Check gas pressure and tighten tubing			

Source: Clinical Laboratory, Huntington Memorial Hospital, Pasadena, California. Reprinted with permission.

Exhibit 13–6 Orientee Rating Scale Form

Employee Behaviors	*Rating (1, 2, 3, 4, 5)*
Conducts and records systems assessment on all patients on each shift	______
Checks medication record against Kardex at the beginning of each shift	______
Communicates appropriately with charge nurse and other staff	______
Completes all ordered care	______
Administers ordered medications in a timely and accurate manner	______
Communicates significant changes in patients' conditions to physician	______
Transcribes physicians' orders accurately and completely	______
Documents all care performed and all observations made	______
Assesses patients' reactions to illness and hospitalization	______
Encourages patients to express feelings about hospitalization, illness, and recovery	______
Assesses family/friend support system	______
Performs teaching necessary for patient and family to cope with discharge	______
Calls appropriate resources to aid in patient/family adjustments	______

Number Values

1 Clearly unacceptable performance; actions show incomplete assessment of situations and consistent poor judgment. Care performed late, incompletely, or inaccurately. Charting inadequate.

2 Borderline performance; actions inconsistent, with frequent errors and unclear planning and use of time. Charting scant and unhelpful to rest of staff.

3 Adequate performance; actions provide for patient safety and well-being, but assessments are incomplete and poorly documented. Little patient/family support or teaching offered. Charting acceptable.

4 Good performance; actions show careful planning and care administration. Patient assessments complete and well documented. Patient/family teaching and support complete and well thought out.

5 Excellent performance; actions uniformly demonstrate superior care with extra details planned and carried out. Unusually good teaching and support with careful evaluation of effectiveness performed. Charting completed in a succinct, detailed manner.

Involving orientees in their own evaluation increases the chances of these three conditions being met. The new information must come from the evaluator, but the motivation to try new behaviors must come from the learner. Constructive evaluation also implies specific suggestions for improvement, which fulfills the third condition. How much more valuable will the alternatives be if the employee helps discover them? The greatest benefit of self-evaluation is that people who are encouraged to evaluate themselves are more likely to develop the habit of self-evaluation and will gradually need less direction from someone else in improving performance.[20]

Exhibit 13–7 is an example of a form encouraging self-evaluation. Designed for new graduates, the questionnaire gives the orientee an opportunity to analyze not

---

Exhibit 13–7 New Graduate Orientation Evaluation

1. What are your strongest skills in nursing?

2. What are your weakest areas in relation to nursing?

3. What skills would you like to improve or master next?

4. Do you feel that being involved with a New Graduate Orientation program was of value to you? Explain.

5. Have you been well received by the nursing staff you are working with?

6. Do you feel comfortable asking questions or asking for help?

7. Are you taking your breaks regularly? Why or why not?

8. How do you feel about working 40 hours per week?

9. What are you doing for fun and relaxation now that you are working full time?

10. State three goals that you would like to accomplish in the next three months:

only performance but attitudes, acceptance, goals, and reactions to the orientation program itself.

REACTIONS TO ORIENTEE EVALUATION

Is evaluation widely practiced, and if so, what is done to deal with identified deficiencies? In an extensive study, Manning surveyed a number of hospitals to discover their evaluation techniques and reactions. Skill checklists and subjective evaluation by an observer were the methods most commonly employed. The method considered most valid by 62 percent of the respondents was observer evaluation, most commonly done by the manager. When deficiencies in knowledge or skills were identified, 65 percent of the units "always" took measures to correct them; 32 percent "usually" did so. Units that attempted to correct deficiencies used a variety of methods: extended orientation periods, extra projects, and additional classes or experiences were required. Only 71 percent of these units reported reviewing the orientee's performance at a later time.[21]

Unless follow-up and continuing feedback occurs, there is no point in evaluating performance in the first place. If the orientee improves, that needs to be expressed. If no improvement is seen, then the orientee should be terminated before becoming a permanent employee. The purpose of the probationary period is to enable the organization and the worker to judge whether or not the employment decision was correct. If either party feels that a mistake has been made, the relationship should end before probation is completed.

CONCLUSION

Orientees should be evaluated before, during, and at the completion of orientation. Although official performance appraisal is the responsibility of managers, orientation instructors must evaluate the participants' grasp of material presented in order to alter teaching strategies and review confusing content. Testing and observation are the two main strategies involved in both classroom and clinical evaluation. The orientees should be encouraged to assess their own performance and participate in finding alternative behaviors if needed.

Chapter 14 will explore methods of evaluating both instructor performance and the impact of the orientation as a whole. Although not the most comfortable of evaluations, assessment of teaching effectiveness and content selection and presentation is more likely to benefit the organization in the long run than group or individual employee evaluation.

NOTES

1. *Webster's Third New International Dictionary of the English Language, Unabridged, 17th Edition* (Chicago: Encyclopedia Britannica, 1976), 786.

2. Helen M. Tobin, Pat S. Yoder-Wise, and Peggy K. Hull, *The Process of Staff Development: Components for Change,* 2d ed. (St. Louis: C.V. Mosby Co., 1979), 162.

3. Em Olivia Bevis, *Curriculum Building in Nursing,* 2d ed. (St. Louis: C.V. Mosby Co., 1978), 192.

4. Laura Mae Douglass and Em Olivia Bevis, *Nursing Leadership in Action* (St. Louis: C.V. Mosby Co., 1974), 55.

5. *Training and Continuing Education: A Handbook for Health Care Institutions* (Chicago: Hospital Research and Educational Trust, 1970), 89.

6. Margaret L. Pohl, *The Teaching Function of the Nursing Practitioner,* 3d ed. (Dubuque, Iowa: Wm. C. Brown Co., 1978), 144.

7. Stuart M. Shaffer, Karen L. Indorato, and Janet A. Deneselya, *Teaching in Schools of Nursing* (St. Louis: C.V. Mosby Co., 1972), 44.

8. Dorothy L. Zufall, "Testing: A Creative Experience for Learners and Educators," *Cross-Reference* 7, no. 2 (March-April 1977): 8.

9. Ascher J. Segall et al., *Systematic Course Design for the Health Fields* (New York: John Wiley and Sons, 1975), B–97.

10. Zufall, "Testing," 9.

11. Harriet L. Schneider, *Evaluation of Nursing Competence* (Boston: Little, Brown & Co., 1979), 116.

12. Zufall, "Testing," 9.

13. Tobin, Yoder-Wise, and Hull, *Staff Development,* 169.

14. Pohl, *The Teaching Function,* 144.

15. Schneider, *Evaluation,* 1.

16. Tobin, Yoder-Wise, and Hull, *Staff Development,* 170.

17. June T. Bailey and Karen E. Claus, *Decision Making in Nursing: Tools for Change* (St. Louis: C.V. Mosby Co., 1975), 106.

18. Tobin, Yoder-Wise, and Hull, *Staff Development,* 170.

19. Wilbert J. McKeachie, "The Role of Faculty Evaluation," *National Forum* 63, no. 2 (Spring 1983): 38.

20. Pohl, *The Teaching Function,* 147.

21. S. Manning, "Characteristics of Burn Orientation Programs," *Journal of Burn Care Review* 4, no. 1 (January-February 1983): 52.

Chapter 14

Program Evaluation

Why evaluate programs and teaching performance? The evaluation process is time consuming and sometimes threatening. Does it yield useful results? The answers to these questions lie in an analysis of just what education is. Education is a means; the ends are self-sufficient people who contribute to our world.[1] The aim of education is to develop useful skills, knowledge, and attitudes in learners that result in positive behavior change.[2] This cannot happen effectively without educators discovering what changes are positive and what methods will bring them about. Evaluation investigates the results of education, leading to change and revision if necessary. This process of investigation can help you answer these questions:

1. Did my actions make a difference?
2. Was it worth the effort?
3. What should be changed to reach the objectives?[3]

Since the goal of all staff development is to change employee behavior in some desired direction, the evaluation must look at results on the job as well as in the classroom. Although this is part of employee evaluation, overall program evaluation looks at the causes of those results. Converting classroom knowledge to on-the-job behavior change requires four factors to be present:

1. There must be commitment on the part of the learner to want to change.
2. The change of behavior must be ego-enhancing.
3. The new behavior must be goal-directed and clearly defined by the objectives.
4. The application of new skills must be fully supported by the organization.[4]

The learner controls the first factor; the manager and the organization control the second and fourth. Only the third is managed by educators. This points up the problem of causation in program evaluation. You can do everything right: identify and measure outcomes of the objectives, report the results to the right people, change the program to accommodate the results—but can you actually demonstrate a causal relationship between the observed changes and the orientation program? How much change was caused by individual intelligence and motivation or managerial and co-worker support? Job performance is strongly affected by work group and organizational expectations and customs; educational effectiveness depends largely on the way the program is supported and reinforced by higher management.[5]

WHO SHOULD EVALUATE?

Evaluation is not a one-department process, let alone a one-person one. A number of people should be involved in evaluating orientation, including orientees, staff members, managers, administrators, committees, instructors, and clients. Tobin, Yoder-Wise, and Hull caution that there should always be specific reasons for asking a person to participate in evaluation.[6] To this might be added the point that any person who does participate deserves some sort of feedback on the results of that participation.

Such reporting of results should be planned when evaluation is first being developed, so that a method of disseminating results is built into the process. Besides communicating the evaluation findings to the various people and committees who need to know them, be sure that any program changes made in response to evaluation are also communicated. If no action is ever taken on evaluation results, it is better to eliminate the costly and time-consuming process altogether.

THE EVALUATION PROCESS

Yourman feels that orientation has two purposes:

1. To acquaint new employees with facts about work, the work environment, relationships, and opportunities;
2. To acquaint managers with the employees' potentials, limitations, aspirations, and attitudes.

Therefore, the fundamental measurements of an orientation program should be employee performance, growth, and morale.[7] How can such reactions be evaluated? The problem is not so much finding information as deciding what information to look for—you must limit data gathering to avoid being inundated.

There are two kinds of evaluation: formative and summative. *Formative* evaluation takes place while the program is in progress to determine how to reach goals set at the beginning. The primary reason for formative evaluation is to furnish feedback to the system as an ongoing process so that any needed changes can be made to achieve the objectives.[8] *Summative* evaluation determines how well the final goals were actually met at the end of the program. Kaufman and Thomas recommend paying special attention to these questions:

1. Did the program really make a difference?
2. Did the program meet and fulfill the objectives?
3. Were the gaps identified in the needs assessment filled?
4. Are the students performing at the level specified in the goals statements?[9]

Both formative and summative evaluation can be analyzed one of four ways:

Reaction—measuring the responses of participants to the program and the instructor.
Learning—measuring the acquisition of knowledge.
Behavior—measuring the change in skills occurring as a result of training.
Results—measuring the organizational effects of training.[10]

Student Reaction

Measuring participant reaction to orientation is easy and results in immediately usable information, but it is extremely subjective. Although learner feedback helps identify which teaching methods are effective for a given group, the personalities of the instructor and the orientees greatly affect such feedback. Evaluations of instructor performance often bear little relation to the program objectives; they are very likely to be expressions of personal prejudice, either positive or negative.[11]

Since learner reaction forms are unlikely to be discontinued, how can they be constructed to provide useful information about teaching performance?

1. Determine what you want participants to react to (content, instructor, methods of presentation, facilities, etc.).
2. Compose a comment sheet containing these factors.
3. Encourage written comments to explain or amplify reactions.[12]

There is disagreement over whether or not evaluations of teacher performance should be anonymous. Some feel that participants will be afraid to give critical feedback if they can be identified. Anyone who has watched an angry instructor scrutinize handwriting in an attempt to identify the author of a negative evaluation can appreciate the force of that argument. On the other hand, since instructors must document and substantiate their evaluations of learners, why shouldn't the same requirement be made for teacher evaluations? Carpenito and Duespohl feel that criticism takes a different and often more constructive form when the authors must identify themselves.[13] An uneasy compromise is sometimes achieved by making signatures optional.

Another controversy with respect to reaction forms concerns rating scales and open-ended questions. Exhibit 14–1 shows a typical rating scale form, on which participants are asked to rank their reactions from one to five, with five representing excellent performance. The advantage to this type of form is ease of compilation—the results can be summarized and quickly reported. The drawback, however, is that this form makes it all too easy merely to scribble in numbers with no clarification. If all fives are received, what exactly made the program so satisfying? If all ones appear, what went wrong? And if, as is often the case, a safe middle ground of threes and fours result, does that give the instructor any kind of useful feedback? This kind of form must include space for additional comments, and the instructor should encourage participants to use that space.

An open-ended format promotes more helpful feedback by asking questions that must be answered in more detail. Exhibit 14–2 shows such a form requesting information about content and presentation, but without direct questions about the instructor. This reduces threat and focuses participants on areas that can be improved, rather than on the teacher's personality. The advantage in using this sort of form is the amount of useful information that can be elicited from an involved group. The disadvantage is that someone uninterested in commenting on the program can choose to leave it blank or jot down a hasty "well done" or "okay."

Exhibit 14–3 shows an evaluation form specifically for orientation. Administered at the end of the program, it seeks to elicit usable feedback about the program content and organization through a mix of check-off and open-ended questions. When thoughtfully completed it can provide enormously useful information; hastily or inadequately answered it is worthless.

Exhibit 14–4 is an evaluation for a new graduate program that again is an amalgam of rating-scale and open-ended comments. Each session contained within the seminars is included for evaluation. The results can be shared with the presenters and plans for change incorporated into the next program. Generally, it is wise not to make sweeping changes based on the reactions of one group; validate those opinions with at least one more group unless you feel strongly that the first participants were right.

Some instructors argue that learner reactions should not be used at all, since new employees may have difficulty identifying what should or should not be taught in orientation. This "teacher knows best" philosophy is appealing, since our area of expertise is education and no one really enjoys being evaluated. But are learner

Exhibit 14–1 Program Reaction Sheet

Program ______________________ Date ____________

Section I: Please answer the following questions on a scale of 1-5 with 5 = Excellent job, 4 = Good job, 3 = Average job, 2 = Fair job, and 1 = Poor job.

Question	Rating	Comments
1. Did the program meet the prestated objectives?		
2. Was the program as a whole presented at your level of understanding?		
3. Was the program presented in an interesting manner?		
4. Was the day and time convenient?		
5. Was the program presented in a way that you will be able to use the information personally and/or professionally?		

Section II: Please rate the information presented from 1-5 with 5 = Excellent, 4 = Good, 3 = Average, 2 = Fair, and 1 = Poor.

Topic	Organization of Presentation	Adequacy of Time to Cover the Material	Increased Your Knowledge	Questions Answered to Your Satisfaction	Comments
1.					
2.					
3.					

Section III: Use reverse side for further suggestions and comments.

Source: Education Department, Huntington Memorial Hospital, Pasadena, California. Reprinted with permission.

Exhibit 14–2 Open-Ended Evaluation Form

PARTICIPANT REACTION FORM

COURSE TITLE: ______________________ DATE: ____________

1. WHAT DID YOU LIKE MOST ABOUT THE PROGRAM?

____

____

____

2. HOW WOULD YOU IMPROVE THE COURSE?

____

____

____

____

3. HOW WILL YOU USE THIS INFORMATION?

____

____

____

____

4. WOULD YOU ADVISE YOUR PEERS TO ATTEND THIS CLASS? YES [ ] NO [ ]

5. COMMENTS: ______________________________

____

____

____

NAME ______________________________
(OPTIONAL)

Source: Education Department, Huntington Memorial Hospital, Pasadena, California. Reprinted with permission.

Exhibit 14–3 Orientation Evaluation Form

1. Do you feel you had a working knowledge of hospital policies and procedures by the end of Orientation classes?
   ____ No ____ Yes
   How could you have learned more?
   ____
   ____
   ____
2. Did the Orientation classes help you adjust to your unit and individual work situation?
   ____ No, not at all ____ They were some help ____ They helped a great deal
   What would have helped your adjustment?
   ____
   ____
   ____
3. What part of your Orientation classes did you find most helpful? Why? __________
   ____
   ____
   ____
4. What part did you find least helpful? Why? ____________________
   ____
   ____
   ____
5. Was the Orientation folder you were given helpful to you?
   ____ No, not at all ____ It helped a little ____ It was very helpful
   What would you like to see included or left out of it? ________________
   ____
   ____
   ____
6. What would you suggest to make the orientation classes more helpful to you and other orientees? ________________________________
   ____
   ____
   ____
   ____
   ____
   ____
   ____
   ____

Source: Education Department, Huntington Memorial Hospital, Pasadena, California. Reprinted with permission.

reactions truly so useless? Cohen located studies of validity involving 68 courses in university settings and found an overall validity coefficient of .4 between mean student ratings and mean achievement. This leads Cohen to believe that student ratings are probably the best single source of information about whether or not students are learning from a teacher, other than measures of actual achievement.[14]

Exhibit 14–4 New Graduate Orientation Evaluation

Please evaluate the seminar presentations. These forms are anonymous, so please be frank.

Group warm-up exercise
Continue to use in program? Yes ____ No ____
Comments: ______________________________

Use the following code to rank the seminar sessions:

1 = useful
2 = fair
3 = not useful

Reality Shock ________ Comments: ______________________________

Consumer Tips on CE ________ Comments: ______________________________

Laboratory Services Tour ________ Comments: ______________________________

Night Shift ________ Comments: ______________________________

Communication Styles ________ Comments: ______________________________

Enterostomal Therapy ________ Comments: ______________________________

Intravenous Review ________ Comments: ______________________________

Leadership Styles ________ Comments: ______________________________

Patient Education ________ Comments: ______________________________

Code Blue Review ________ Comments: ______________________________

Overall, did you feel the seminars were a productive use of time?

What were the beneficial aspects of the program?

Exhibit 14–4 continued

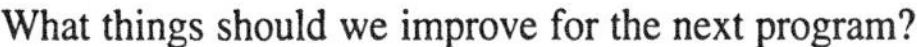

What things should we improve for the next program?

If a good friend (who just happened to be a senior nursing student) asked you about the new graduate orientation program here, what would you tell her/him?

Source: Education Department, Huntington Memorial Hospital, Pasadena, California. Reprinted with permission.

Self-Evaluation by the Instructor

Validate learner reactions with your own observations and reactions to the program. Most instructors have a good feel for how well the session went and how much was communicated to the students. Was there enough time to cover what was planned? If not, a different organization of content may be necessary, or some objectives may even have to be eliminated. How was the rapport and communication between teacher and group members? Did the participants seem involved and interested, or did their body language indicate boredom? Did you elicit feedback at frequent intervals to ensure that the content was being assimilated? Was a mix of teaching strategies used?

Pohl suggests developing the habit of making mental notes about what is happening during a teaching session for later consideration. Each session should be analyzed as soon as possible, and written notes made if the evaluation must be delayed.[15] Such a set procedure of self-assessment promotes continued improvement of teaching as you become more conscious of the effects certain actions have on the participants.

Peer Evaluation

Having another instructor observe and evaluate your teaching can be disconcerting, but if the observer is a trusted and respected colleague the experience can prove helpful. The arrangement should be reciprocal, with instructors taking turns observing each other's classes. Shaffer, Indorato, and Deneselya recommend that supervised teaching be conducted without administrative ratings, so that all concerned understand that the primary objective of the endeavor is to provide constructive criticism of both positive and negative aspects of the observed performance.[16]

Dennis et al. report a procedure developed by nursing department faculty in a university. All instructors met together to plan the peer evaluation system, identifying three categories of achievement: (1) presentation, style, and strategy; (2) student-teacher climate; and (3) knowledge. Members felt that the degree of behavior manifested was not what should be evaluated, but rather whether it was done or not. Specific behavior descriptions were prepared for each category, and the group agreed that each faculty member would be evaluated at least once a semester. The completed form is given to the person being evaluated.[17]

Some research findings show peer observations to have low reliability.[18] It is probably better to have other instructors help judge the content and organization and orientees assess what impact the instructor has had on them. The teacher can then personally weigh his or her own perceptions of the experience against the feedback offered by students and peers.

Learning

Assessment of learning has already been described in Chapter 13. Measurement through the pretest/post-test process can determine changes in knowledge caused by exposure to orientation content. Remember that increases in learning do not necessarily transfer over into clinical practice.

Behavior

Measuring performance is usually more objective and more acceptable to adults than testing; it also improves communication with line managers, since the units provide the data.[19] Chapter 13 dealt with the technique of observation as a method of employee evaluation. The results of orientee evaluations should also help assess the effectiveness of the program. During unit rounds, talk with managers and preceptors about new employee performance. Are content areas being used on the job? Can the orientees recall and apply the information they received in class? Is there a performance deficit that has shown up in a number of new people? If so, more emphasis in that area may be required.

Observation of performance, especially over a period of time, is the most effective method for determining the worth of a program.[20] If the orientation objectives translate into behaviors exhibited on the unit, the program is achieving its main aim—preparing new employees to work productively and effectively.

Results

The most significant and difficult kind of evaluation concerns the organizational benefits derived from orientation. Results evaluation involves a cost versus benefit analysis, where benefits include such desired outcomes as reduced costs, improved productivity, reduction of turnover and absenteeism, fewer accidents, and improved patient care.[21] Results such as these are affected by so many different factors that it is almost impossible to relate the program directly to them. But the effort to do so is worth it, for what better way to justify our programs—and our jobs—than by showing a positive return on investment.

All the methods used in the initial needs assessment described in Chapter 2 now must be used again to validate the fact that some change has taken place. Interviews and survey questionnaires elicit opinions from key organizational people about the perceived results of the program. How has performance changed since the first data collection? Audits, quality assurance reports, and incident/accident reports provide factual data about the quality of patient care. Employee accident reports can show whether or not the safety and body mechanics portions of orientation are having an impact. When compared with previous reports, all of these sources can indicate improvement through new content added to the program.

The personnel department is a valuable source of data on such organizational indices as turnover, performance evaluations, and exit interviews. The staffing office or individual departments keep records of absenteeism and tardiness. Some departments even have measures of individual productivity that can be used for evaluation purposes.

How can you actually prove that the program makes a difference? The only way is to construct an experimental design in which randomly assigned participants exposed to the orientation program are compared with randomly assigned participants in a control group. Any changes in learning, behavior, or results demonstrated by the experimental group and not by the control group could legitimately be claimed as a result of orientation. In most settings this is impractical, as well as unfair to new employees. Yet the findings of this kind of evaluation can be startling. In one study, a total of six groups of nurse interns and their matched controls who did not participate in the intern program were followed over a three-year period. The evaluation model considered the effects of the internship on such variables as clinical competence, role transition, job satisfaction, perceived autonomy, job turnover, and career patterns. Preliminary data collected in the first year revealed few significant differences between the intern and control groups. The most striking difference was in the scores on the role transition questionnaire. The results seemed to indicate that the control group made a significantly better adjustment to the staff nurse role.[22]

No evaluator wants to encounter such results in evaluation. An unforeseen result is disappointing and frustrating. On the other hand, isn't it better to discover some ineffective part of the program and either change or eliminate it rather than continuing to devote time, money, and other resources to something that is not accomplishing the objectives?

REVISING ORIENTATION

Revision of content, organization, and approach is a constant process. Just as there is no such thing as the perfect program, you will never bring orientation to a point where you are completely satisfied with it. Revision should be based on the findings of evaluation: reaction, learning, behavior, and results. Changes based on data gathered from orientees, staff, and managers give them a feeling of ownership in the program, so be sure to communicate such changes when they are made.

It is best to make minor changes in response to convincing feedback when it occurs but schedule regular reassessment of the entire program periodically. If this is done once a year or every six months (or whatever interval seems appropriate in your situation), new ideas from staff feedback, assessment techniques, or administrative mandates can be piloted, evaluated, and made part of the program.

Another source for revisions is professional reading and contacts with other educators. Books and journal articles contain different approaches that can spark a new way of looking at an old problem. Meeting with orientation instructors from other institutions at workshops, conventions, and meetings of such organizations as the American Society of Healthcare Education and Training (ASHET) and the American Society of Training and Development (ASTD) leads to idea sharing that can save time and money—a new method of self-study, an instructional game, different forms.

CONCLUSION

Program evaluation is much more difficult than participant evaluation. Formative assessment throughout the program and summative assessment at the end must be based on the overall objectives. To conduct an evaluation we can examine reactions, learning, behavior, and results. Of these, the results analysis of the program's impact on the organization is both very hard to accomplish and potentially very beneficial. The greatest problem with organizational evaluation concerns determining causation—program impact can be claimed only if an experimental design utilizing control groups is used. Feedback from evaluation determines program revision, a planned process that should be scheduled at least once a year.

When planning any major changes in orientation, the entire needs assessment process should be recycled, particularly the interviews with hospital decision makers. Putting such people on notice that you are striving to update orientation and maintain practice at a high level is an excellent method of remaining organizationally visible.

NOTES

1. Roger Kaufman and Susan Thomas, *Evaluation Without Fear* (New York: New Viewpoints, A Division of Franklin Watts, 1980), 29.
2. Ibid., 29.
3. Ibid.
4. J. Sterling Livingston, "New Trends in Applied Management Development," *Training and Development Journal* 37, no 1 (January 1983): 20.
5. S. Dale McLemore and Richard J. Hill, *Management Training Effectiveness* (Austin, Tex.: Bureau of Business Research, The University of Texas, 1965), 7.
6. Helen M. Tobin, Pat S. Yoder-Wise, and Peggy K. Hull, *The Process of Staff Development: Components for Change*, 2d ed. (St. Louis: C.V. Mosby Co., 1979), 168.
7. Julius Yourman, "Orientation of New Employees," in *Improving the Effectiveness of Hospital Management*, ed. Addison C. Bennett (New York: Metromedia Analearn, 1972), 264.
8. Em Olivia Bevis, *Curriculum Building in Nursing*, 2d ed. (St. Louis: C.V. Mosby Co., 1978), 291.
9. Kaufman and Thomas, *Evaluation Without Fear*, 112.
10. John W. Newstrom, "Employee Training and Development," *Encyclopedia of Professional Management* (New York: McGraw-Hill Book Co., 1978), 291.
11. *Training and Continuing Development: A Handbook for Health Care Institutions* (Chicago: Hospital Research and Educational Trust, 1970), 251.
12. Donald L. Kirkpatrick, "Management Development and Training," *Encyclopedia of Professional Management* (New York: McGraw-Hill Book Co., 1978), 295.
13. Lynda Juall Carpenito and T. Audean Duespohl, *A Guide for Effective Clinical Instruction* (Wakefield, Mass.: Nursing Resources, 1981), 157.
14. Wilbert J. McKeachie, "The Role of Faculty Evaluation," *National Forum* 63 no. 2 (Spring 1983): 37–38.
15. Margaret L. Pohl, *The Teaching Function of the Nursing Practitioner*, 3d ed. (Dubuque, Iowa: Wm. C. Brown Co., 1978), 145.
16. Stuart M. Shaffer, Karen L. Indorato, and Janet A. Deneselya, *Teaching in Schools of Nursing* (St. Louis: C.V. Mosby Co., 1972), 54.
17. Connie M. Dennis et al., "Peer Evaluation: A Process of Development," *Journal of Nursing Education* 22, no. 2 (February 1983): 94–95.
18. McKeachie, "Faculty Evaluation," 38.
19. John Dopyera and Louise Pitone, "Decision Points in Planning the Evaluation of Training," *Training and Development Journal* 37, no. 5 (May 1983): 67–68.
20. Tobin, Yoder-Wise, and Hull, *Staff Development*, 174.
21. Kirkpatrick, "Management Development," 296.
22. Lillian K. Gibbons and Dana Lewison, "Nursing Internships: A Tri-State Survey and Model for Evaluation," *Journal of Nursing Administration* 10, no. 2 (February 1980): 34–36.

Part V

Future Trends in Orientation

Chapter 15

Issues and Directions

What does the future hold for orientation and those who teach it? As hospital costs increase and controls clamp down ever tighter, how can we ensure that tight budgetary restrictions won't turn back the clock to the days when new employees were simply deposited at their work station and told to "go to it"? Not only do the new employees deserve better—so do the patients.

Orientation is perhaps the most costly function in the education department in terms of expended manpower hours.[1] In a 1975 study, the total national cost of hospital orientation was estimated to be $135 million, 60 percent of the total national cost of $226 million for all hospital education—and these calculations were made only on the basis of direct salary components of costs for instructors and participants.[2] A more recent study discovered that the median costs for orientation were $796 per nurse for hospitals in the 6–99 bed category and $1,501 per nurse for hospitals in the 300+ bed category.[3]

Given these figures, how can orientation programs be justified to administration—and to the consumers who are footing the bills? Educators must attack this problem from three directions: (1) cost-effectiveness analysis, (2) new needs for hospital orientation, and (3) new methods of orientation delivery.

COST-EFFECTIVENESS ANALYSIS

Analyzing Program Costs

Hospital administrators are business executives, and businesspeople like to have figures when making decisions. Gone are the days when educators could blithely assume that orientation would automatically be approved because it's "good." It may be good, but what has it done for the hospital lately? And exactly what does it cost? If you don't know the exact costs of your program, find out now.

Each program should be analyzed in terms of what it costs to produce and present, as well as evaluate. How many hours did each instructor put in developing the class (research, arranging for rooms and refreshments, composing handouts, etc.)? How many hours were actually spent in class? At first these are painful figures to contemplate. All those hours put in just to prepare one class? Don't be discouraged if this initial step indicates that you spent many hours of preparation for every hour of class. The classic training rule is that every hour of classroom instruction requires *40 hours* of instructor preparation.[4]

To those hours should be added any time spent on follow-up: putting away equipment, reading completed assignments or classwork, grading tests, completing records, etc. Add preparation hours to class hours and hours spent on follow-up and multiply the total by the instructor's hourly salary. Add to that any time spent by anyone else involved in the class: other instructors, the secretary who did the typing, the audio-visual technician who videotaped something, etc.

Now calculate the costs of the materials you used. How much did the film cost, or the transparencies, or the slides? Divide that total cost by the number of times you expect to be able to use this item and you have the cost of a single showing. What were the costs for photocopying the syllabus, handouts, case studies, and tests? Multiply the number of copies by the cost per copy and you'll know.

Take the attendance sheet and note the categories of employees who were in the class: RN, pharmacist, unit secretary, physical therapist, etc. Build in a mechanism for discovering who attended on their own time—have a space to check on the roll sheet or a box on the application form. Anyone who was not paid to attend is not added to the cost. But all participants attending on paid time are part of the cost analysis, and orientation is a required class where everyone is paid to attend. Multiply the relevant hourly salaries (personnel department can give you average hourly salaries for each category of employee) by the class hours and add them all together to get the cost to the institution for those people to participate.

Put in any other program costs such as consultant fees, workbooks, refreshments, etc., and add all these figures together to find out the total cost of the course. To be completely accurate, you would have to calculate overhead costs such as depreciation on the building, carpeting, equipment, etc., but this figure is hard to come by and generally will not affect the final total to a considerable degree. At this point the total cost per class looks appallingly large enough—how can it be justified?

Analyzing Program Benefits

There is another part to the equation—the results or benefits derived from the class. DelBueno and Kelly have developed a method of comparing descriptive outcomes with costs in order to determine the cost effectiveness of educational programs. They feel that "a cost-effective staff development department is one that achieves maximum desirable results or outcomes at a minimum expenditure of resources."[5]

Learning outcomes range from attendance only (the participants were there and breathing, but that's all you can say for sure) to consistent on-the-job performance without external reinforcement, calculated on a 1 to 5 scale. This data can be obtained only by observation and follow-up during and after class. If most participants can pass a written test the class achieved a 2, if they successfully complete a simulated problem in class a 3, if they apply content to actual work situations with reinforcement from another person a 4, and so on. Costs are also ranged from 1 to 5 using dollar amounts in a scalar relationship. Then the two figures are related as a ratio, with effectiveness as the first number and cost as the second. Studies using this system discovered an outcome for staff nurse orientation of 3:2.75, and for allied orientation of 3:2. This would imply that the benefits of orientation at that particular hospital outweigh the costs.[6]

Another method of calculating benefits versus costs was used by McKenzie. Course participants in a medical terminology class were interviewed six weeks after the course concluded and asked to estimate the amount of time saved each day as a result of taking the class. The cost of conducting the program for 17 employees was estimated at $3,373.14. Because participants did not have to use the dictionary to look up terms, the mean number of hours saved per year was 130.3, and the estimated mean number of years of future service was 2.63. Gross cost benefits for 2.63 years were estimated to be $25,749.65. The total estimated costs were subtracted from the estimated cost benefits, rendering a net benefit estimate of $22,376.55.[7]

Whatever cost-effectiveness measurement system you use, remember that education is difficult to quantify. People can disagree with your methods or results despite your best efforts, and there are some educational benefits that are impossible to measure—or sometimes even identify. Rosenthal describes the "ceremonial effects" of training, where training motivates employees to higher performance levels because it fosters inclusion, facilitates commitment to organization goals, and demonstrates the organization's willingness to invest in its employees. Employees feel that the organization cares about them and wants to contribute to their growth and development. These serendipitous effects are associated with the act of training itself, not the content.[8]

Imagine trying to measure such effects! When claiming the less easily quantifiable benefits, it may help to review the findings of formal studies performed across the nation. As far back as 1956, Weber found that good orientation programs serve to enrich jobs and increase satisfaction with them.[9] Kearsley states that inadequate training of employees typically results in increased overtime, high turnover, poor morale, the need for additional employees, and excessive equipment maintenance.[10]

When presenting such findings to administration, stress the fact that 70 percent of a hospital's operating budget goes to payroll costs.[11] With such a tremendous investment already committed to employees, it only makes sense to develop them to the greatest extent possible. If new employees leave soon after hire because of inadequate orientation, the hospital suffers a double penalty of recruitment/induction costs and an overworked staff more likely themselves to terminate employment. The last word on this subject has really been said by McKenzie, who stated: "All things considered, it seems that what really costs is the absence of hospital education."[12]

ELICITING ADMINISTRATIVE SUPPORT

When presenting a proposal for revising or expanding the orientation program, be sure to plan your strategy carefully. Research the professional literature. What has been tried and how has it worked? Use these facts to back up your proposal. Visit hospitals in the area and find out what community practice is. If other programs are more extensive than yours, stress the need to bring orientation up to competitive standards. If other orientations are limited, point out how an excellent, coordinated program will increase hospital prestige in the community and help recruitment.

Conduct a formal needs analysis, using the procedures described in Chapter 2. The better you know the institution's problems (which often are symptoms of learning needs), the more prepared you will be to construct the proposal for the program. Make it a formal document with a problem statement, alternative actions, proposed solution, short- and long-range objectives, required budget, and procedure for evaluation. Your presentation must be aimed at eliciting commitment and support from key administrative personnel.

Another selling point not to be overlooked is finding techniques that will reduce the hours spent by educators during orientation. Self-study components generally decrease costs, as will be discussed in the section on new methods of orientation delivery. Hebert identified some other strategies to cut down on instructor time:

1. Identify departmental developers who can function as partners with new employees (in the absence of formal preceptor programs) and assist them in becoming acquainted with the hospital and their departments.
2. Prepare information packets containing facts about each department, which new employees can study when they have a chance.[13]

NEW NEEDS FOR HOSPITAL ORIENTATION

Another aspect of justifying orientation's existence involves the new needs appearing in hospitals. As in the past when institutions moved from orienting only nurses to orienting all employees, now more and more organizations are presenting induction programs to such diverse groups as physicians, agency nurses, volunteers, and students.

Physician Orientation

All too often, new house staff are given a brief welcoming speech by the chief of staff and then deposited on the units to learn the ropes from harried senior physicians or equally harried nurses. If an organized program is presented, the new doctors will not only function better, they will also feel more a part of the organization. Content of the program should be worked out between the medical staff and the education department, since both areas will be involved in implementation. Once the program objectives are agreed on (what do you want the new physicians to be able to do upon completion?), content selection should be relatively easy. Some areas that might be covered include:

1. Orientation to the physical plant (tours, maps, etc.).
2. Review of the organizational structure of both the medical section and the rest of the institution.
3. Introduction to key people (for example, administrators, the director of nursing and nursing supervisors, head nurses and other department heads who interface with house staff). This can be accomplished in a formal meeting or at a luncheon or wine and cheese party where everyone is introduced and then can mingle and get to know one another in a social atmosphere.
4. Policies and procedures relating to the medical staff: What must be included in a written order? Are verbal orders allowed? Is a "Do Not Resuscitate" order acceptable? What must be included in the admission history and physical? What are the routine preoperative orders? The number of things that new physicians need to know right away is staggering.
5. The folkways of the institution: Is a certain type of clothing expected for different levels of medical staff? What are the expectations when a house staff physician is on call? These and other unwritten rules need to be communicated to the new doctors before they begin work.

Lawnwood Medical Center in Fort Pierce, Florida, prepared a 25-page booklet for new house staff members. The booklet contained the center's history; administration's organization, philosophy, and policies; a list of each department's hours and services, and a staff directory. New physicians receive the booklet, a tour, and explanations of policies and procedures, accompanied by chart reviews. Feedback from the house staff has been overwhelmingly positive.[14]

Reeder, Moran, and Connolly describe a two-and-one-half day workshop for medical students coming into the operating room. The OR educators spoke with attending physicians and residents to discover what needs and frustrations they encountered when they were beginning medical students. Based on this input a syllabus was formulated with course objectives, an outline, and examples of various forms—order sheets, care plans, assessment forms, etc. The workshop oriented the medical students to the basic clinical and technical skills necessary to function in the area. All participants agreed that fellow medical students would benefit from similar presentations.[15]

Agency Nurses

Many hospitals rely on independent agencies, sometimes called registries, to supply supplemental staff when needed. Controversy surrounds this approach, its supporters citing cost savings by being able to adjust staffing according to the census, its detractors claiming that "rent-a-nurses" who come in for a day and leave destroy continuity of care, as well as personal and professional accountability. These and other arguments are likely to continue, since the use of registry nurses remains necessary for many institutions.

One of the gravest problems connected with the use of agency nurses lies in their orientation, or rather the lack of it. In too many instances these nurses come in to a hospital they have never seen before, receive little or no information, and are expected to carry a full patient load. Horror stories are told of registry nurses being placed in charge of units with no preparation. One of these concerned a registered nurse and two nurse attendants who were assigned to care for a 16-patient unit on the day shift; there was no unit secretary, no charge nurse—and none of the three agency people had ever seen the hospital before! No one told them where equipment was kept, how charting should be done, or how to order or charge anything.

There is no excuse for this sort of dangerous situation. JCAH clearly states: "Prior to their performing nursing functions within a patient care area, nursing personnel who are not hospital employees must be provided any required orientation by the nursing department/service."[16] Regulations aside, common sense and concern for patient safety dictate that nurses new to the hospital should receive a briefing on policies and procedures.

Of 159 hospitals responding to a questionnaire, 78 percent reported that they require agency nurses to be oriented to emergency procedures, location of supplies, and unit routine. Time spent varied from 15 minutes to 40 hours; the average was 8 hours. Some respondents said content was covered by giving reading material to the supplementary nurses; others covered it in the classroom.[17]

Another study used actual observers rather than questionnaires. On every shift, in every hospital in the sample, the observers noted that no one reviewed the nurse's responsibilities or defined terms used on the unit to registry nurses. Of the hospitals studied, 38 percent regularly used registry nurses as charge nurses. In 72 percent of the hospitals, registry nurses were expected to start working even though they lacked understanding of the hospital's philosophy of care or knowledge of the location of supplies, emergency equipment, or diagnostic departments.[18]

Two different studies with differing results—one where the hospitals reported their practices, the other where actual practice was noted by independent observers. Obviously, procedures vary from hospital to hospital, but some mechanism must be built into each hospital's system to orient temporary employees.

Some hospitals require orientation instructors to spend 30 minutes or so with a new registry nurse, giving quick instructions on the institution's methods and requirements of care delivery. While effective, this one-on-one approach is costly and proves impractical on a daily basis. Other organizations provide long orientations for agency personnel on a periodic basis, not accepting anyone for duty who has not attended one of the sessions.

At the University of California's Irvine Medical Center agency nurses receive an orientation checklist from a series designed for registered nurses, licensed vocational nurses, and nurse attendants. The charge nurse on the unit takes responsibility for orientation. At the end of the day another form is used to evaluate the temporary nurse's performance, and a decision is made about whether or not to allow the nurse to work at the medical center again.[19]

All of these approaches have their advantages and their drawbacks. One way of incorporating several features would be to prepare an instruction booklet containing directions on how to transcribe orders, chart, record medications, and any other procedures or policies the nurse needs to know. Unit personnel could then give agency workers a quick tour and explanation of the assignment and expectations, and the booklet would be available to review the nurse's role and clear up later questions. Exhibit 15–1 shows an excerpt from such a booklet. A pocket size format (perhaps three inches by five inches) would be especially convenient, and could be kept by agency nurses for reuse when they returned to the hospital.

The only sure thing about approaches to agency nurse orientation is that something must be done. If your hospital has no current system in place, take the initiative and develop one. Having nurses entirely uninformed about hospital policies and procedures is unsafe and inexcusable.

Exhibit 15–1 Excerpt from Registry Orientation Book

Medication Administration Procedure

1. Check Medication Administration Record (MAR) for each patient against Kardex. Settle any discrepancies by checking original order.
2. Intravenous solutions and piggybacks are delivered premixed and stored in the refrigerator. Check bottle number and label accuracy against MAR before administration. Note time on tearoff label, initial label, and drop it in the green box marked "Pharmacy."
3. When administering medications, take the entire cart into the patient's room—never leave it unattended.
4. Insulin and heparin dosages must be doublechecked by another licensed nurse, who then initials the record along with the nurse administering the medication.
5. Check drug, dosage, route, and time when pouring the medications—before, during, and after. When ready to administer, ask the patient's name and check the wristband ID. *Do not* rely on room number, bed card, or verbal check alone. The only definitive identification is the wristband—it must *always* be checked.
6. Remain in the room until all medications are taken. Never leave any drug at the bedside unless a physician ordered one of the following drugs for self-administration: topical ointments, birth control pills, nitroglycerin tablets, or antacids. There must be a written order for any of these, and no other drug is allowed at the bedside, with or without an order.
7. To record medication administration, draw a diagonal line through the printed hour and initial it. Be sure your full signature is at the proper date and shift at the bottom of the page.

Volunteer Orientation

Volunteers perform many vital functions for hospitals. Their dedication and selflessness deserve not only recognition but a proper orientation to the institution. The program may be given by the public affairs department or by a special volunteer department, but in many hospitals the education department is either responsible for the presentation or else helps teach part of it.

Since volunteers raise large sums of money for the hospital as well as provide free service, the program generally has special touches lacking in more routine orientations. Award luncheons, professionally prepared booklets, service pins, even designer uniforms—all of these have been used for volunteer programs. In this sort of atmosphere, the learning objectives must include public relations aspects as well as straight educational ones. The history of the hospital might stress the long heritage of quality care provided to the community, and a review of administrative personnel might be done at a brunch, luncheon, or tea where the volunteers meet and mingle with the administration.

One of the most important areas to cover is the volunteer's role in the organization. What are the things they can or cannot do? Most hospitals do not allow nonemployees to deliver any direct patient care. Duties are often limited to working at the information desk, the gift shop, and the waiting rooms, or to delivering flowers, gifts, or library carts. If volunteers are allowed to perform patient care they should be taught exactly how each task must be done. For instance, if volunteers are allowed to discharge patients, they need to know how to safely operate a wheelchair—lock adjustment, safe entrance and exit from elevators, the policy on leaving a patient unattended, etc.

Junior volunteers are high school age people who work during the summer and occasionally on weekends. These volunteers may be considering a career in health care, so it behooves us to encourage and support them. The more involved they become in hospital activities, the more informed a decision they can make later on. Junior volunteers often learn bedmaking, wheelchair safety, even how to feed patients. Acting as junior nurse attendants, they will be allowed to make unoccupied beds, assist with ambulation, pick up trays, and perform other simple patient care duties. This should be attempted only when the nursing staff is able to provide constant supervision.

Externships

Recently, a new approach to combating reality shock has come to light: in a number of hospitals student nurses work during summer break as externs. Although students have often worked as nurse attendants for extra money, extern programs attempt to provide not only clinical experience but an actual taste of staff nurse roles and responsibilities.

These programs vary greatly, but a typical plan might be to pay the student nurses who have the required clinical experience (generally a minimum of junior year level) a nurse attendant salary. Performing bedside care and gradually working up to a full patient load, the externs have the opportunity to observe various nurses give care, team lead, and take charge of the unit. Although not permitted to perform those tasks themselves, externs see the problems and pressures firsthand, as well as a good view of how nurses cope on a daily basis. Some hospitals even provide observations in surgery and other specialty units.

Arlington Hospital in Virginia started an externship program for third-year baccalaureate students in 1978. Students may choose to practice in medical-surgical areas, operating room, obstetrics, or psychiatric nursing. Receiving both classroom and on-the-job experience, each extern is paired with a registered nurse who has volunteered to act as preceptor. In return for participating in the program at the nurse attendant salary, students sign an agreement that they will work for the hospital for one year after graduation. Arlington has discovered considerable savings when these nurses become permanent staff members; an extern graduate needs only one week of orientation classes and two weeks of clinical experience, whereas an ordinary new graduate requires one week in the classroom and a minimum of four weeks of clinical experience.[20]

NEW METHODS OF ORIENTATION DELIVERY

Individualized Study

The trend in orientation is definitely moving away from the classroom and toward a self-study approach. Several self-study programs have been described in previous chapters. Before changing your entire presentation to self-study, however, it is a good idea to consider a gradual transition starting with an initial pilot program. The information covered in the safety section of orientation seems easily converted to self-study because it is fairly clear cut, with sharply defined guidelines. Whatever content is chosen for the first self-study program, careful pre- and post-testing should be conducted, so results from the pilot can tell you whether the particular student population learns effectively with this approach.

Computer Assisted Instruction

Computer Assisted Instruction (CAI) refers to the direct use of the computer for the facilitation and certification of learning.[21] Computer learning was discussed in Chapter 4 as a teaching strategy, but its profound future impact on hospital education needs to be explored. Developments in both hardware (the computer, display terminals, printers, disk drives) and software (authoring languages, operating systems, programs) make CAI far more sophisticated than the old programmed learning with straight progression of limited questions and answers. Today's technology provides such things as multiple branches for different levels of answers, increased interaction with complex responses between learner and computer, and graphic displays that make it possible to portray such things as ECG patterns.

Hospitals tend to shy away from computers not so much from inherent conservatism as from concern about potential costs. These systems are not cheap. Although hardware costs are most visible, the development of courseware represents the largest cost component of a CAI system. CAI courseware requires on the order of 100 to 400 hours of development time for every hour of instruction produced.[22]

On the plus side, employees have been shown to produce greater on-the-job performance as a result of CAI in comparison with conventional classroom approaches.[23] Use of CAI can result in reduced training time, another potential area of savings. And perhaps most important of all, CAI produces computer literacy in employees. Kearsley feels that given the increasing prevalence of computer systems in modern society and the workplace, ability to comfortably interact with computers is quickly becoming a basic life-coping skill.[24]

Some instructors fear CAI because "it will take away my job." Nothing could be further from the truth. Developing computer programs for education requires special training. Once instructors are taught how to write courseware (a service usually provided by the company installing the system), they become specialists whose expertise is highly valued. No one else in the institution will know how to develop and program CAI presentations, so the education experts are vital to all operations. Instructors can even market their services to other institutions. In fact, one way to make a computer system more affordable is for several hospitals to share services, either at the time of purchase or on a rental basis.

Centralized Versus Decentralized Orientation

Traditionally, hospitals have split education into nursing inservice education and non-nursing education. Nursing programs were conducted by instructors working in the department of nursing and all other programs were taught in individual areas such as respiratory therapy, pharmacy, housekeeping, etc. Today many institutions are decentralizing their management systems to bring decision making down to the lowest level possible. Doesn't a decentralized education process fit right into this growing trend?

Unfortunately, in practice decentralization of education leads to waste, miscommunication, and duplication of services. Rostowsky found that decentralization in a hospital's nursing service organizational structure achieved staff satisfaction and major improvements in patient care—except in the area of education. After further evaluation, the hospital established a separate department of education and charged it with the responsibility of meeting the total hospital's educational needs.[25] A number of hospitals have established similar departments. It will be interesting to see the long-range results of these programs.

Collum suggested that centralized hospital education is more relevant and beneficial. Gaps and shortcomings have occurred when nursing inservice education has been isolated. Establishing hospitalwide education departments results in specially prepared, better qualified instructional resources, better coordination, better use of educational materials, and increased staff members' growth through their integration into the hospital's total operation.[26]

If a centralized education department has the responsibility of providing orientation for all hospital employees, the programs will be coordinated to minimize repetition of information—and to prevent vital data from "falling through the cracks" as people move through the system. Although clinical follow-up and reinforcement must be done in the individual areas, central coordination promotes closer communication and support for orientees and preceptors alike.

Grubb feels that the trend toward centralizing the responsibility for managing hospital education and training will accelerate. This will make the education function less subject to the stultifying factors of professional and organizational "turf" disputes that inhibit hospitals from optimally using their most valuable asset—their human resources.[27]

CONCLUSION

Future directions in orientation include an increasing need for demonstrating cost effectiveness to administration; actively eliciting administrative support for the program; discovering new needs for orientation in such diverse groups as physicians, agency nurses, volunteers, and students; and developing new methods and philosophies of education delivery, including self-study, computer assisted instruction, and a centralized approach to orientation for all hospital employees.

The responsibility for orienting new employees to the hospital environment requires instructors to study trends and stay current with professional developments, health care discoveries, and the forces of change within hospitals and society. The orientation instructor can have a significant impact on health care practice and quality patient care, which is cause for both pride and concern. Pride in one's ability and expertise and concern for maintaining and increasing both—these lead instructors on a never-ending quest for new information. May it always be so.

NOTES

1. Caryl G. Hebert, "Orientation," in *Hospital-Based Education,* ed. Corinne B. Linton and James W. Truelove (New York: Arco Publishing, 1980), 60.

2. Howard S. Rowland and Beatrice L. Rowland, *Nursing Administration Handbook* (Rockville, Md.: Aspen Systems Corp., 1980), 179.

3. Marjorie Beyers et al., "Results of the Nursing Personnel Survey, Part I: RN Recruitment and Orientation," *The Journal of Nursing Administration* 22, no. 4 (April 1983): 36.

4. Edward McCabe, "The High Cost of Training," *Health Care Education* 7, no. 6 (October-November 1978): 8.

5. Dorothy J. delBueno and Karen J. Kelly, "How Cost-Effective Is Your Staff Development Program?" *Nurse Educator* 5, no. 5 (September-October 1980): 12.

6. Ibid., 14–17.

7. Leon McKenzie, "Hospital Education—Does It Cost Too Much?" *Cross-Reference* 7, no. 2 (March-April 1977): 7.

8. Steven M. Rosenthal and Bob Mezoff, "Improving the Cost/Benefit of Management Training," *Training and Development Journal* 34, no. 12 (December 1980): 102–104.

9. Helen J. Weber, "Aspects of Job Satisfaction Through Orientation and Inservice Programs," *Hospital Progress* 37, no. 12 (December 1956): 63–64.

10. Greg Kearsley, *Costs, Benefits, and Productivity in Training Systems* (Reading, Mass.: Addison-Wesley Publishing Co., 1982), 58.

11. Julius Yourman, "Orientation of New Employees," in *Improving the Effectiveness of Hospital Management,* ed. Addison C. Bennett (New York: Metromedia Analearn, 1972), 235.

12. McKenzie, "Hospital Education," 8.

13. Hebert, "Orientation," 60.

14. "Nurse Wrote the Book on M.D. Orientation," *R.N. Magazine* 46, no. 4 (April 1983): 124D.

15. Jean M. Reeder, Margaret L. Moran, and Mary S. Connolly, "A Nursing Workshop for Medical Students," *AORN Journal* 36, no. 1 (July 1982): 119–128.

16. *Accreditation Manual for Hospitals, 1983 Edition* (Chicago: Joint Commission on Accreditation of Hospitals, 1983), 120.

17. Patricia A. Prescott et al., "Supplemental Nursing Services: How and Why Are They Used?" *American Journal of Nursing* 83, no. 4 (April 1983): 557.

18. Genevieve M. Clavreul and Sue Caviness, "Unsafe Nursing Practices and What You Can Do About Them," *Nursing Life* 2, no. 3 (May/June 1983): 42–43.

19. "When In Doubt, Orient Agency Nurses," *R.N. Magazine* 46, no. 4 (April 1983): 32C.

20. Mary C. Johnson, "An Externship in OR Nursing," *AORN Journal* 36, no. 2 (August 1982): 260–266.

21. Robert L. Burke, *CAI Sourcebook* (Englewood Cliffs, N.J.: Prentice-Hall, 1982), 16.

22. Kearsley, *Costs, Benefits, and Productivity,* 159.

23. Ibid., 173.

24. Ibid., 174.

25. R.D. Rostowsky, "Beneficial By-Products of Decentralization," *Hospital Topics* 58, no. 1 (January-February 1980): 7–8.

26. E.W. Collum, "Bring Nurse Education Out of Isolation," *Hospitals* 54 (June 16, 1980): 195–198.

27. Allen W. Grubb, "Roles, Relevance, Costs of Hospital Education and Training Debated," *Hospitals* 55 (April 1, 1981): 79.

Bibliography

Archbold, Carl R. "Our Nurse-Interns Are a Sound Investment." *R.N. Magazine* 40 (September 1977): 105–112.

Armstrong, Myrna L. "Bridging the Gap Between Graduation and Employment." *Journal of Nursing Administration* 4 (November-December 1974): 42–48.

Armstrong, Myrna L., Marjorie King, and Barbara Miller. "Avoiding Orientation Burnout." *Nursing Management* 13 (July 1982): 24–27.

Bachman, David J. "Orientation for the New OR Nurse." *AORN Journal* 31 (February 1980): 199–212.

Bayley, Elizabeth W., and Anne W. Ravreby. "Development of Competency-Based Orientation for Burn Nursing." *Journal of Burn Care Review* 4 (January/February 1983): 36–55.

Bell, Deanne French. "Assessing Educational Needs: Advantages and Disadvantages of Eighteen Techniques." *Nurse Educator* 3 (September/October 1978): 15–21.

Benner, Patricia. "Issues in Competency-Based Testing." *Nursing Outlook* 30 (May 1982): 303–309.

Bittel, Lester R. *What Every Supervisor Should Know,* 3d ed. New York: McGraw-Hill Book Co., 1974.

Bowen, Barbara J. "An Orientation Program in a Small Hospital." *Supervisor Nurse* 9 (February 1978): 25–30.

Chagares, Robin Isaak. "The Nurse Internship Question Revisited." *Supervisor Nurse* 11 (November 1980): 22–24.

Chapman, Thelma. "Orientation—First Impressions Last." *The Journal of Continuing Education in Nursing* 6 (January-February 1975): 44–47.

Charron, Denise C. "Save the New Graduate." *Nursing Management* 13 (November 1982): 45–46.

Copeland, Winifred L., and Barbara E. Miller. "Development of a Modular Curriculum for Nursing Service Orientation." *The Journal of Continuing Education in Nursing* 7 (July-August 1976): 10–15.

Crockett, Judy. "Restructuring an Orientation Program for Nurses Utilizing Management By Objectives Principles." *The Journal of Continuing Education in Nursing* 9 (March-April 1978): 19–21.

Cronin-Stubbs, Diane, and Patricia S. Gregor. "Adjustment of the New Graduate to the World of Nursing Service." In *Teaching Tomorrow's Nurse: A Nurse Educator Reader,* edited by Susan Mirin. Wakefield, Mass.: Nursing Resources, 1980.

deHamel, M., and J.A. Peitchinis. "Increasing Competence of Newly Hired Nurses." *Dimensions in Health Service* 52 (July 1975): 40.

delBueno, Dorothy J. "Accountability: Words and Action in Inservice Education." *Washington State Journal of Nursing* 47 (Summer 1975): 8–9.

delBueno, Dorothy J., and Marjorie C. Quaife. "Special Orientation Units Pay Off." *American Journal of Nursing* 76 (October 1976): 1629–1631.

Dell, Mary Swope, and Ethel Griffith. "A Preceptor Program for Nurses' Clinical Orientation." *Journal of Nursing Administration* 7 (January 1977): 37–38.

Demers, Patricia M. "Developing a Primary Nurse." *Nursing Management* 12 (December 1981): 28–30.

Drum, Randall L., and F. David Cordova. "Analyzing and Developing Effective Instructional Behaviors for Allied Health Educators." *Journal of Allied Health* 8 (November 1979): 226–231.

Dunn, Sally A., and Marge Johnson. "Education of the New Employee: An Orientation Program for Infection Control." *APIC* 7 (September 1977): 9–12.

Farrell, Jane. "Orienting the R.N. in Orthopedics." *The ONA Journal* 4 (April 1977): 91–93.

Feldman, Michael. "Planning for an Indirect Training Style." *Training and Development Journal* 36 (October 1982): 79–81.

Fitzhugh, Zoe-Anne, Rose Morrisey, Margaret Waugh, and Judith A. Kierran. "A Patient-Centered Orientation Program." *Hospitals* 48 (January 16, 1974): 72–78.

Floyd, Gloria Jo, and Billy Don Smith. "Job Enrichment." *Nursing Management* 14 (May 1983): 22–25.

Frank, Betsy Dennis, and Betsy Brockett Powell. "A Skills Checklist for Orientation of Associate Degree Nurses." *Supervisor Nurse* 6 (May 1975): 39–45.

Furlong, Beth. "Setting the Stage for Learning." *American Journal of Nursing* 82 (February 1982): 300–301.

Gahart, Betty L. "Employee Orientation Is a Whole New Ball Game." *Hospital Forum* 18 (March 1975): 5–6.

Ganong, Joan M., and Warren L. Ganong. *Nursing Management,* 2d ed. Rockville, Md.: Aspen Systems Corporation, 1980.

Gelbach, Deborah L. "Designing the Training Room of Your Dreams." *Training* 19 (December 1982): 16–21.

Georgenson, David L. "The Problem of Transfer Calls for Partnership." *Training and Development Journal* 36 (October 1982): 75–78.

Gibb, Peter. "The Facilitative Trainer." *Training and Development Journal* 36 (July 1982): 14–19.

Gold, Leon. "Job Instruction: Four Steps to Success." *Training and Development Journal* 35 (September 1981): 28–32.

Guida, Frances Kyner. "Treating the Orientation Overload System." *Supervisor Nurse* 8 (October 1977): 28–31.

Hahn, Margot, and Kathleen Magill. "A Bridge Over Troubled Waters." *The Journal of Continuing Education in Nursing* 4 (May-June 1973): 15–19.

Hammerstad, Susan Miller, Suzanne Hall Johnson, and Linda Vireno Land. "New Graduate Orientation Program." *The Journal of Continuing Education in Nursing* 8 (July-August 1977): 5–11.

Hanson, Shirley M.H. "Role Orientation and Integration." *The Journal of Continuing Education in Nursing* 7 (November-December 1976): 23–26.

Harrell, Joanne R. Summey. "Orienting the Experienced Critical Care Nurse." *Supervisor Nurse* 11 (January 1980): 32–33.

Hartin, Jean M. "Nursing Apprenticeship." *Nursing Management* 14 (March 1983): 28–29.

Harty, Lawrence D., and Bruce P. Monroe. *Objectives for Instructional Programs*. Orange, Calif.: Insgroup, 1975.

Hilliard, Mildred. *Orientation and Evaluation of the Professional Nurse*. St Louis: C.V. Mosby Co., 1974.

Huntsman, Ann J. "Self-Paced Learning Requires Careful Planning." *Cross-Reference* 7 (March-April 1977): 1–3.

Infante, Mary Sue. *The Clinical Laboratory in Nursing*. New York: John Wiley and Sons, 1975.

Jackle, Mary, Carolyn Ceronsky, and Joan Peterson. "Nursing Students' Experience in Critical Care: Implications for Staff Development." *Heart and Lung* 6 (July-August 1977): 685–690.

Jung, Steven M. "Third Party Validation of Training Effectiveness." *Training and Development Journal* 37 (March 1983): 6–7.

Kachelmeyer, Pat. "Registered Nurse/Licensed Practical Nurse Orientation Program." *The Journal of Continuing Education in Nursing* 6 (May-June 1975): 40–47.

Keaveny, Mary E. "Needed: Better Orientation for A.D. Graduates." *Nursing '73* 3 (July 1973): 52–53.

Kibbee, Priscilla. "Developing a Model for Implementation of an Evaluation Component in an Orientation Program." *The Journal of Continuing Education in Nursing* 11 (September-October 1980): 25–29.

Knauss, Parry J. "Staff Nurse Preceptorship: An Experiment for Graduate Nurse Orientation." *The Journal of Continuing Education in Nursing* 11 (September-October 1980): 44–46.

Kramer, Marlene. *Reality Shock: Why Nurses Leave Nursing*. St. Louis: C.V. Mosby Co., 1974.

Leffler, Margaret. "A Hospital Orientation Program for Agency Nurses." *Supervisor Nurse* 10 (August 1979): 46–50.

Littlejohn, Carolyn E. "What New Staff Learned and Didn't Learn." *Nursing Outlook* 28 (January 1980): 32–35.

Lunn, Sharon. "Evaluation: A Critical But Neglected Step in Education Design." *AORN Journal* 37 (January 1983): 94–98.

Martin, Patricia D. "The Graduate Nurse Transition Program." *Supervisor Nurse* 7 (December 1976): 18–22.

Meisenhelder, Janice Bell. "A First Hand View of the Unit Teacher Role." *Journal of Nursing Administration* 12 (January 1982): 35–39.

Morgan, Dorothy. "Upgrading the Work of New Graduate Nurses." *Dimensions in Health Service* 55 (November 1978): 28–33.

Morris, Lona, Linda Girch Hitchcock, Joan Kucera, and Karen Vernon. "Student-Made, Student-Played Games." *American Journal of Nursing* 80 (October 1980): 1816–1818.

Newstrom, John W., and Melissa S. Leifer. "Triple Perceptions of the Trainer: Strategies for Change." *Training and Development Journal* 36 (November 1982): 91–96.

Nixon, Kathleen, and Merla Russell. "Creating a Learning Environment." *Canadian Nurse* 71 (November 1976): 24–26.

Orleck, Carol. "Transition: Student to Practitioner." *Nursing Management* 13 (January 1982): 23–24.

Page, Gordon G. "Written Simulation in Nursing." *Journal of Nursing Education* 17 (April 1978): 28–32.

Patterson, Judith R. "Get New Employees Off to a Good Start!" *MLO* 9 (November 1977): 111–114.

Peitchinis, Jacquelyn. "Orientation Programs and the Competent Nurse." *Dimensions in Health Service* 55 (June 1978): 12–13.

Pohutsky, Lorraine. "An Orientation Plan for Nurses." *Supervisor Nurse* 10 (October 1979): 23–26.

Ponthieu, J.F. "Gaining Mutual Independence Through Training." *Supervisory Management* 27 (April 1982): 16–19.

Rantz, Marilyn J. "A Modular Approach to Unit Orientation." *Supervisor Nurse* 11 (June 1980): 48–51.

Roland, Naomi. "Planning an Orientation Course." *Nursing Mirror* 145 (June 12, 1975): 63–65.

Romines, Jack A., and Bill Crump. "A Self-Examination for Training Developers." *Training and Development Journal* 36 (July 1982): 76–80.

Rosenberg, Mac. J. "The ABCs of Instructional Systems Design." *Training and Development Journal* 36 (October 1982): 44–50.

Sanford, Nancy D. "Teaching Strategies for Inservice and Staff Development Educators." *The Journal of Continuing Education in Nursing* 10 (November-December 1979): 5–10.

Schmalenberg, Claudia, and Marlene Kramer. "Bicultural Training: A Cost-Effective Program." *Journal of Nursing Administration* 9 (December 1979): 10–16.

Schmidt, Martha C., and Marjorie C. Quaife. "Orientation by Contract." *Supervisor Nurse* 5 (October 1974): 38–44.

Seigel, Harriet. "Innovations in Orientation: A Community Health Learning Package." *Journal of Nursing Education* 21 (May 1982): 8–15.

Smith, Carol E. "Planning, Implementing, and Evaluating Learning Experiences for Adults." *Nurse Educator* 3 (November-December 1978): 31–39.

Smith, Robert M. *Learning How To Learn: Applied Theory for Adults*. Chicago: Follett Publishing Co., 1982.

Smith, Roger F. "How To Link Theory and Practice in Training Courses." *Radiography* 48 (March 1982): 47–57.

Stopera, Virginia, and Donna Scully. "A Staff Development Model." *Nursing Outlook* 22 (June 1974): 390–393.

Tesla, Angie. "Training Our Own Replacements." *AORN Journal* 26 (August 1977): 382–388.

Tisone, Carmella L. "Orientation of the New R.N." *Hospital Topics* 54 (July/August 1976): 12–15.

Tobin, Helen M. ''Orientation Programs for New Nurses.'' *AORN Journal* 28 (November 1978): 952–966.

Turnbull, Ellie. ''Rewards in Nursing: The Case of Nurse Preceptors.'' *Journal of Nursing Administration* 13 (January 1983): 10–13.

Waddell, Geneva. ''Simulation: Balancing the Pros and Cons.'' *Training and Development Journal* 36 (January 1982): 80–83.

Weintraub, Joan M. ''Program Integrates O.R. Professional Nurses' Needs.'' *AORN Journal* 28 (September 1978): 512–524.

West, Nat, Joan Sudbury, and Mitch Ayers. ''An Objective Appraisal Instrument for Registered Nurses.'' *Supervisor Nurse* 10 (March 1979): 32–38.

Williams, Shirley. ''An Inactive Nurse Returns to Work.'' *Nursing Management* 12 (November 1981): 44–48.

Zemke, Ron, and Susan Zemke. ''Thirty Things We Know for Sure About Adult Learning.'' In *Adult Learning in Your Classroom,* edited by Philip G. Jones. Minneapolis: Training Books, 1982.

Zielstorff, Rita Deziel. ''Orienting Personnel to Automated Systems.'' *Journal of Nursing Administration* 6 (March-April 1976): 14–16.

Index

Note: Page numbers in *italic* indicate entry is found in artwork.

D

J

L

M

N

R

S

T

U

V

W

Y

Z

About the Author

Ann Haggard is currently the Management Development Coordinator for Huntington Memorial Hospital in Pasadena, California. Before taking charge of the development activities for all hospital managers, she was the Orientation Coordinator, handling the centralized nursing orientation. Besides serving as secretary for the southern California chapter of the American Society of Healthcare Education and Training, she also belongs to the American Society of Training and Development and the Inservice and Health Education Council of Los Angeles. Dr. Haggard's publications concern hospital management, nursing education, and staff development. She has been a nursing instructor, inservice director, head nurse, and a staff nurse. Her educational background includes degrees from Michael Reese Hospital and Medical Center School of Nursing (R.N.), Pittsburgh State University (B.S.N.), California State University-Los Angeles (M.S.), and Columbia Pacific University (Ph.D.). She is a member of the national Phi Kappa Phi Honor Society.